Atlas of
Oral and Maxillofacial
Surgical Instruments

Atlas of
Oral and Maxillofacial
Surgical Instruments

Syed Ahmed MDS

Professor and Head, and PG guide
Department of Oral and Maxillofacial Surgery, and Ex-Principal
MIDSR Dental College, Latur, Maharashtra

Ex-Professor and Head, and PG guide
Department of Oral and Maxillofacial Surgery, and Ex-Principal
Al-Badar Dental College, Gulbarga

Consultant Oral and Maxillofacial Surgeon
Sahara Accident Hospital and Alfa Superspecialty Hospital, Latur

Sheeraz Badal MDS

Associate Professor and PG guide
MIDSR Dental College, Latur

Consultant Oral and Maxillofacial Surgeon
Panhale Dentofacial and Implantology Hospital and Sandikar Orthopaedic and Trauma Hospital
Latur, Maharashtra

Sandesh Chougule

Resident, Department of Oral and Maxillofacial Surgery
MIDSR Dental College
Latur, Maharashtra

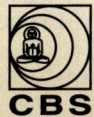

CBS

CBS Publishers & Distributors Pvt Ltd

New Delhi • Bengaluru • Chennai • Kochi • Kolkata • Mumbai
Hyderabad • Jharkhand • Nagpur • Patna • Pune • Uttarakhand

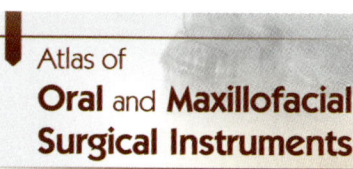

Atlas of
Oral and **Maxillofacial**
Surgical Instruments

ISBN: 978-93-86478-12-2

Copyright © Authors and Publisher

First Edition: 2017

Published by Satish Kumar Jain and produced by Varun Jain for

CBS Publishers & Distributors Pvt Ltd

4819/XI Prahlad Street, 24 Ansari Road, Daryaganj, New Delhi 110 002, India.
Ph: 23289259, 23266861, 23266867 Website: www.cbspd.com
Fax: 011-23243014   e-mail: delhi@cbspd.com; cbspubs@airtelmail.in.
Corporate Office: 204 FIE, Industrial Area, Patparganj, Delhi 110 092
Ph: 4934 4934   Fax: 4934 4935   e-mail: publishing@cbspd.com; publicity@cbspd.com

Branches

- **Bengaluru:** Seema House 2975, 17th Cross, K.R. Road,
  Banasankari 2nd Stage, Bengaluru 560 070, Karnataka
  Ph: +91-80-26771678/79   Fax: +91-80-26771680   e-mail: bangalore@cbspd.com

- **Chennai:** 7, Subbaraya Street, Shenoy Nagar, Chennai 600 030, Tamil Nadu
  Ph: +91-44-26680620, 26681266   Fax: +91-44-42032115   e-mail: chennai@cbspd.com

- **Kochi:** Ashana House, No. 39/1904, AM Thomas Road, Valanjambalam,
  Ernakulam 682 016, Kochi, Kerala
  Ph: +91-484-4059061-65   Fax: +91-484-4059065   e-mail: kochi@cbspd.com

- **Kolkata:** 6/B, Ground Floor, Rameswar Shaw Road, Kolkata-700 014, West Bengal
  Ph: +91-33-22891126, 22891127, 22891128   e-mail: kolkata@cbspd.com

- **Mumbai:** 83-C, Dr E Moses Road, Worli, Mumbai-400018, Maharashtra
  Ph: +91-22-24902340/41   Fax: +91-22-24902342   e-mail: mumbai@cbspd.com

Representatives

- **Hyderabad** 0-9885175004 - **Jharkhand** 0-9811541605 - **Nagpur** 0-9021734563
- **Patna** 0-9334159340 - **Pune** 0-9623451994 - **Uttarakhand** 0-9716462459

Printed at Nutech Print Services, Faridabad, India

Foreword

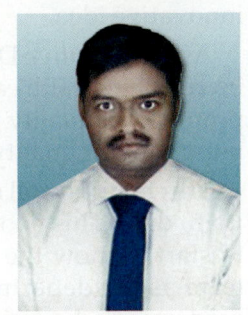

It gives me immense pleasure to write a Foreword to this *Atlas*. This book by Dr Syed Ahmed, *Atlas of Oral and Maxillofacial Surgical Instruments*, is a tour de force. It is well organized, well written, well referenced, and up to date. This book has 14 chapters written by the author and various contributors. There are more than 200 illustrations of surgical instruments, which are remarkable with clear description of each instrument.

The author has to be congratulated for writing an extraordinary book with tireless efforts. The ultimate beneficiaries of the ideas expressed in this book, of course, are the dental, medical, and Ayurvedic faculty interested in surgical practice. This book should be of great interest to the oral and maxillofacial surgeons, craniofacial surgeons, neurosurgeons, otolaryngologists, and postgraduate and undergraduate students.

Dr Syed Ahmed is Professor and Head, and PG guide, Department of Oral and Maxillofacial Surgery, MIDSR, under MUHS. He was also Principal of MIDSR Dental College and Hospital, Latur.

His work as administrator as well as in the academics is highly appreciated and recognized. I wish him "all the best" for this excellent project. I hope the readers can be inspired to take this knowledge, learn it well and then extend it further, for the benefit of mankind.

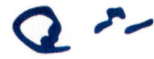

Kalidas D Chavan
Officiating Registrar
Maharashtra University of Health Sciences
Nashik, Maharashtra

Foreword

This book by Dr Syed Ahmed and his colleagues, *Atlas of Oral and Maxillofacial Surgical Instruments*, is a good and innovative idea.

As an Executive Director of MAEER's Pune, Latur campus, I am involved in health care and social activities for 26 years as well as promoter of quality value based medical education which is very important for quality care of the patients.

This book is well organized, well written, well referenced and up to date. This book is "a beginning" for any surgical specialty to start. I know the author Dr Syed Ahmed personally and his team as the department is a part of the institution and their appreciable clinical, academic and administrative work. The ultimate beneficiaries will be the students, doctors, and finally the patients and their relatives.

This book is of great interest to craniofacial surgeons, oral and maxillofacial surgeons, neurosurgeons, otolaryngologists, and others who care for craniofacial and head and neck surgeries.

I congratulate the team and team effort to bring out this extraordinary book.

Shri Ramesh K Karad
Executive Director
MIMSR Campus, Latur

Contributors

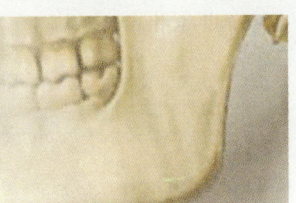

Ahtesham Ahmad MDS
Associate Professor
Deptt of Oral and Maxillofacial Surgery
MIDSR Dental College, Latur, Maharashtra, India
General Surgery Instruments

Alka Sherkhane
Resident, Deptt of Oral and Maxillofacial Surgery
Sighngad Dental College, Pune, Maharashtra, India
Introduction

Amol Doiphode MDS
Associate Professor
Deptt of Oral and Maxillofacial Surgery
MIDSR Dental College, Latur, Maharashtra, India
Tracheostomy Instruments

Arunachaleshwar Balkunde MDS
Assistant Professor
Deptt of Oral and Maxillofacial Surgery
MIDSR Dental College, Latur, Maharashtra, India
Dental Implants Instruments

Ashish Satpute
Resident, Deptt of Oral and Maxillofacial Surgery
MIDSR Dental College, Latur, Maharashtra, India
*Advanced Instruments in Oral and Maxillofacial
Surgery*

Deepak Motwani MDS
Professor
CSMSS College of Dental Science
Aurangabad, Maharashtra, India
Sterilization of Surgical Instruments

Fatima K Shaikh MBBS
Ambejogai, Maharashtra, India
*Classification of Oral and Maxillofacial Surgical
Instruments*

Girish Thakur MS ENT
Vice Principal, Associate Professor and Head
Deptt of ENT
GMC, Latur, Maharashtra, India
Tracheostomy Instruments

Gopal Nagargoje
Resident, Deptt of Oral and Maxillofacial Surgery
MIDSR Dental College, Latur, Maharashtra, India
Sterilization of Surgical Instruments

Hanumant T Karad MS
Professor and Head
Deptt of Ophthalmology
MIMSR Medical College
Latur, Maharashtra, India
General Surgery Instruments

Jeevan Khatri MDS
Professor and Head
Deptt of Orthodontics
CSMSS College of Dental Science
Aurangabad, Maharashtra
Orthognathic Instruments

K Kartiken Reddy MDS
Assistant Professor
Deptt of Oral and Maxillofacial Surgery
Meghna Institute of Dental Sciences
Nizamabad, Telangana, India
Sterilization of Surgical Instruments

Kiran Raddar MDS
Associate Professor
Deptt of Oral and Maxillofacial Surgery
SDM Dharwad Dental College and Hospital
Karnataka, India
Sterilization of Surgical Instruments

M Ehtaihsham MDS
Professor, Deptt of Oral and Maxillofacial Surgery
Vydehi Institute of Medical and Dental Sciences
Bangalore, Karnataka, India
Orthognathic Instruments

Mohammad Yaseen MCh Plastic Surgeon
Professor
Aligarh Muslim University, Aligarh (UP), India
Cleft Lip and Palate Instruments

M Suresh Kumar MDS
Professor and Head
Deptt of Oral and Maxillofacial Surgery
Meghna Institute of Dental Sciences
Nizamabad, Telangana, India
History of Surgical Instruments and Legends

M Veerabhau MDS
Professor and Head
Deptt of Oral and Maxillofacial Surgery
Ragas Dental College, Chennai, Tamil Nadu, India
Maxillofacial Trauma Instrument

■ **Murali Mohan** MDS
Principal
Government Dental College, Vijayawada
Andhra Pradesh, India
Orthognathic Surgery Instruments

■ **Paul V Joseph** MDS, FDRCS
Consultant Oral and Maxillofacial Surgeon
Kochi, Kerala, India
Maxillofacial Trauma Instrument

■ **Priyanka Samel**
Resident, Deptt of Oral and Maxillofacial Surgery
MIDSR Dental College, Latur, Maharashtra, India
Cleft Lip and Palate Instruments

■ **Priyanka Tapsale**
Resident, Deptt of Oral and Maxillofacial Surgery
MIDSR Dental College, Latur, Maharashtra, India
Classification of Oral and Maxillofacial Surgical Instruments

■ **Rahul Lature** MDS
Professor
Deptt of Oral and Maxillofacial Surgery
MIDSR Dental College and Hospital
Latur, Maharashtra, India
Classification of Oral and Maxillofacial Surgical Instruments

■ **Sameer Shaikh**
Resident, Deptt of Oral and Maxillofacial Surgery
MIDSR Dental College, Latur, Maharashtra, India
Rhinoplasty Instruments

■ **Sandesh Chougule**
Resident, Deptt of Oral and Maxillofacial Surgery
MIDSR Dental College, Latur, Maharashtra, India
Exodontia and Minor Oral Surgical Instruments

■ **Sanjay S Byakode** MDS
Associate Professor
Deptt of Oral and Maxillofacial Surgery
Bharati Vidyapeeth Deemed University
Sangli, Maharashtra, India
General Surgery Instruments

■ **Sara Ahmed** 1st Year MBBS
MIMSR Medical College, Latur, Maharashtra, India
Tracheostomy Instruments

■ **SC Bhoyar** MDS
Dean Faculty MUHS Nashik
Dean, Professor and Head
Deptt of Oral and Maxillofacial Surgery
CSMSS Dental College and Hospital
Kanchanwadi, Aurangabad, Maharashtra, India
Distraction Osteogenesis Instruments

■ **Shameen Sultana** BDS
Manchreal, Telangana, India,
Advanced Instruments in Oral and Maxillofacial Surgery

■ **Sheeraz Badal** MDS
Associate Professor
Deptt of Oral and Maxillofacial Surgery
MIDSR Dental College, Latur, Maharashtra, India.
Exodontia and Minor Oral Surgery Instruments

■ **Shoeb Jendi**
Resident, Deptt of Oral and Maxillofacial Surgery
MIDSR Dental College, Latur, Maharashtra, India
Distraction Osteogenesis Instruments

■ **Shraddha Patil**
Resident, Deptt of Oral and Maxillofacial Surgery
MIDSR Dental College, Latur, Maharashtra, India
Advanced Instruments in Oral and Maxillofacial Surgery Instruments

■ **Suchitra Nagare** MBBS
Executive Medical Director
MAEER'S MIT, Talegaon Dhabade, Maharashtra, India
History of Surgical Instruments and Legend

■ **Sunanda Gaddalay** MDS
Professor and Head
Deptt of Conservative Dentistry & Endodontics
MIDSR Dental College
Latur, Maharashtra, India
History of Surgical Instruments and Legend

■ **Swati Jadhav**
Resident, Deptt of Oral Maxillofacial Surgery
MIDSR Dental College, Latur, Maharashtra, India
Dental Implants Instruments

■ **Syed Ahmed Mohiuddin** MDS
Professor and Head
Deptt of Oral and Maxillofacial Surgery
MIDSR Dental College, Latur, Maharashtra, India
Email: drsyedahmed28@yahoo.com
History of Surgical Instruments and Legend

■ **Virendra Ghaisas** MS. ENT
Executive Director, Hospital Administration
MAEER'S MIT
Talegaon Dhabade, Maharashtra, India
Rhinoplasty Instruments

■ **Vithal Lahane** MCh Plastic Surgeon
Consultant Plastic Surgeon, Lahane Hospital
Dinanath Nagar, Savewadi, Latur, Maharashtra, India
Cleft Lip and Palate Instruments

Preface

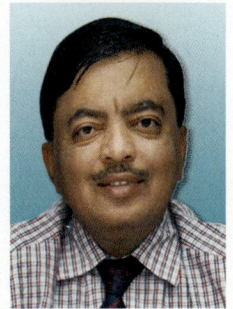

A good surgical result will definitely depend on the precise use of instruments in different surgical procedures. It helps in reducing operating time and surgical morbidity on both hard and soft tissues. A good surgeon grows with experience and experience develops with time and use of appropriate surgical instruments when indicated.

All teachers at the surgical speciality start teaching the difference between a needle holder and hemostat and we grow to understand other instruments that are used for various procedures. Instruments developed from stone age, wood sticks, metals, and now computers and robots are replacing the art of surgical skills.

All surgeons should know the correct use, indications and contraindications of basic instruments. As we continue to realize the importance of instruments in oral and maxillofacial surgeries, we gain a better appreciation of the far reaching consequences of our treatment and surgical results.

This book provides a complete insight into various instruments used in oral and maxillofacial region, which will benefit the practising surgeons, trainees, and undergraduate and postgraduate students to better understand the instruments in detail. There are hardly a few books available in literature exclusively covering instruments in oral and maxillofacial surgery. This is one of them.

It is obliviously impossible for any book of this kind to be either complete or remain up to date for a long period of time. Hence, we have put our sincere efforts to make this book almost complete and up to date including the recent advances and the instrument with photographs.

I would like to express my sincere appreciation to peers and contributors, and everyone who has contributed to the understanding of the precise use of instruments.

Also lastly I am thankful to postgraduate trainees at Department of Oral and Maxillofacial Surgery. Their thirst for knowledge, honesty, and obedient nature, all put together, have made this book a constant source of inspiration.

As the primary author of this textbook, I welcome corrections, criticism and suggestions which will definitely be paid attention to and corrected in subsequent editions to come.

Syed Ahmed

Acknowledgements

The book *Atlas of Oral and Maxillofacial Surgical Instruments* represents the work of many dedicated individuals. The contributors to this *Atlas* are professors, readers, senior lecturers, tutors and residents primarily from the Department of Oral and Maxillofacial Surgery, MIDSR Dental College, Latur, Maharashtra. Apart from this there are a few authors from other institutes and faculty who have lent or donated their expertise time to create a comprehensive text.

And most importantly the result of team work from contributors, computer operator and typist has given us this greatest reward in our quality and endeavour. I sincerely thank my family, my wife Dr Nekparveen, and my daughters Miss Sara and Miss Shaheen, for their patience and not disturbing till the project was completed. Our thanks are also extended to Mr YN Arjuna, Senior Vice President—Publishing, Editorial and Publicity, CBS Publishers & Distriburors, New Delhi, who has approved this project, and Mr Sarkar S and Mr Javed Hashmi, CBS Publishers & Distributors Pvt Ltd, Mumbai, for their active cooperation.

On a personal note, I must thank Prof (Dr) Vishwanath Karad, our Founder and Director General of MAEER'S MIT–Pune and Mr Rameshappa Karad, Executive Director of MIMSR, Latur, for permitting us to go with this concept and achieving academic target. A special thanks to Dr Mangesh Tulshiram Karad, Executive Director of MAEER'S MIT, Pune for his appreciation to complete the project. I would also like to thank Mr Vijay Narayan Kale, Chief Librarian of MIMSR Medical College, Latur, for his support in utilizing the library facilities. I would like to extend my thanks to the Director, Mr Shambhu Bachagoudar, and Mr Shrikant Bachagoudar, SK Surgicals, Pune, who have allowed to use photographs of their instruments.

I do remember a few unforgettable people who shaped my life, to name a few of them, Mr Iqbal Ahmed Saradagi MP, Chairman, Al-Badar Dental College and Hospital, Kalaburagi, Karnataka; Dr C Bhasker Rao, ex-Principal, SDM Dental College, Dharwad; Prof (Dr) Balaji, Dr Venugopal, Government Dental College, Kerala; Prof (Dr) Rahmatullah, ex-Principal, Al-Badar Dental College, Gulbarga; and many more who worked and shared my time and knowledge.

And there are many more to be thanked but above all is God, the 'Almighty', who has enlightened our brain and thoughts in this direction.

Syed Ahmed

Contents

Introduction

Syed Ahmed Mohiuddin, Alka Sherkhane

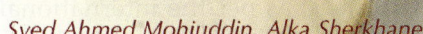

Surgery literally means 'handicraft'. As the ancient derivation of the word indicates, in **Latin, chirurgia** and in **Greek, kheir-ourgos,** or **cheir-ourgos, where kheir/cheir means hand and ourgos means working. Hands and teeth** were the natural 'instruments' that ancient 'Man' used to counter diseases, injuries and any foreign bodies. Gradually instruments made of the organic materials like **bamboo, shell, animal teeth and bones** were invented.

The history of the barber pole is connected with the history of barbers performing elevated work like tooth extraction, bloodletting, administering enemas, and taking care of the wounds along with the customary cutting hair.

Later, as medicine become more defined as a field of its own, efforts were made to separate the academic surgeons from these barber surgeons. In England, barbers were chartered as a guild called the Company of Barbers in 1462 by Edward IV. The surgeons established their own guild 30 years later. Although these two guilds were merged as one by the Statue of Henry VIII in 1540 under the name of United Barber-Surgeons Company in England, they were still separated: Barbers displayed blue and white poles, and were forbidden to carry out surgery except for teeth-pulling and bloodletting; surgeons displayed red and white-striped poles, and were not allowed to shave people or cut their hair. Also, Louis XV of France decreed in 1743 that barbers were not to practice surgery.

The surgeons went on to form a corporation with the title of Masters, Governors and Commonalty of the Honourable Society of the Surgeons in London which was eventually dissolved in 1800 during the reign of George III and replaced by the Royal College of Surgeons.

The instruments used in surgery range from diagnosis to operative ones. The field of medical science has progressed so much that manually used instruments are now replaced by power-driven pieces of equipment that save the time and energy of the surgeon. The modern era of medicine and surgery has paved its way to simplify treatment modalities to derive the outcome out of small effort.

Surgical instruments are the primary need for any kind of surgery that is being performed by a surgeon in his day-to-day life. It forms the backbone of any surgical procedure done for the benefit of the patient. Every surgeon must have a precise and definitive understanding of working mechanism related to every instrument that he uses. If proper knowledge of the instrumentation and their mechanism is lacking, then the operative procedure cannot be efficiently carried out successfully which may lead to more tissue damage, increase the time of operation and does not provide quality service to patients. Today, since more than thousands of instruments are available, it

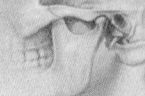

becomes challenging for the beginners in oral and maxillofacial surgery to get acquainted with the application of these instruments in a proper way.

The creative human nature has an ability to search for solution whenever any problem arises. This has led to discovery and invention of new advanced instruments that are simple to use, that can be sterilized, sometime power driven to save the time and provide better quality of service.

This compilation will help dentists, general surgeons, plastic surgeons and oral and maxillofacial surgeons to know about instruments and keep the basic armamentarium in their surgical setup. This will also guide the department involved to organize the instrument as per the international standard, coming home to the expectations of Dental Council of India or Medical Council of India.

"As flute is for musicians, instruments are for surgeons. A best musician plays with best flute; similarly a best surgeon performs with the best instruments."

Chapter 2

History of Surgical Instruments and Legends

Suchitra Nagare, Syed Ahmed Mohiuddin, M Suresh Kumar, Sunanda Gaddalay

"Our Tribute—At a Glance"

MAHARISHI SHUSHRUT (PERIOD 1500 BC)

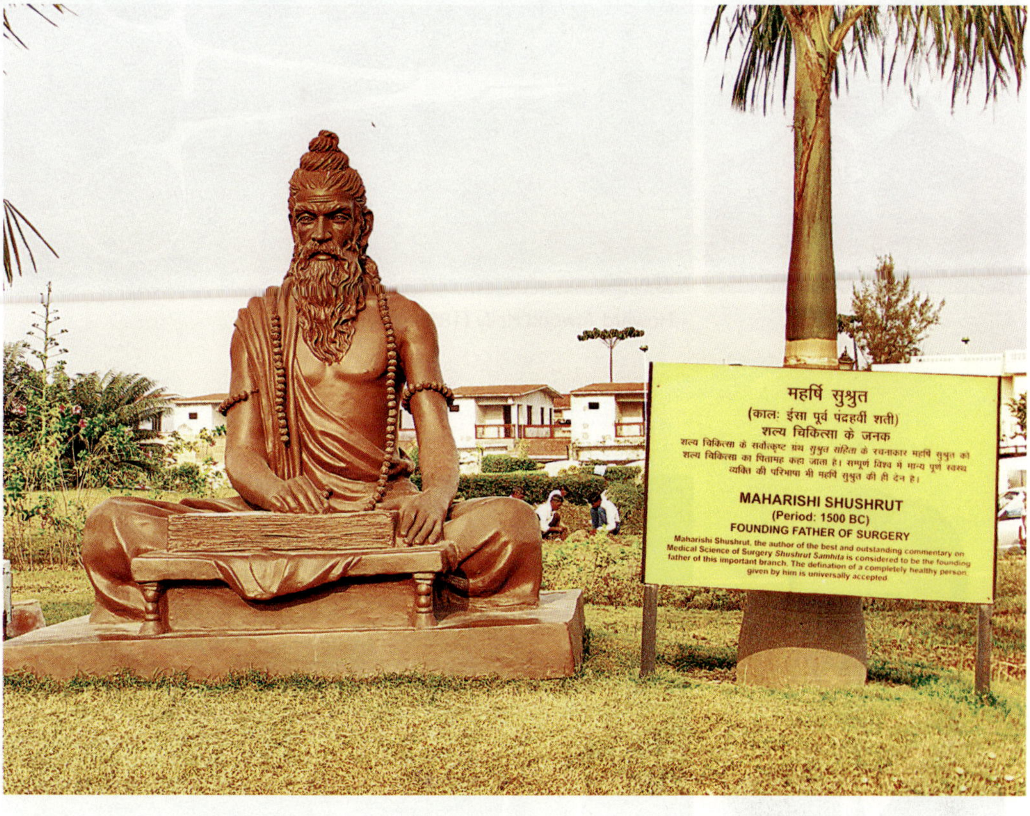

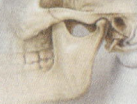

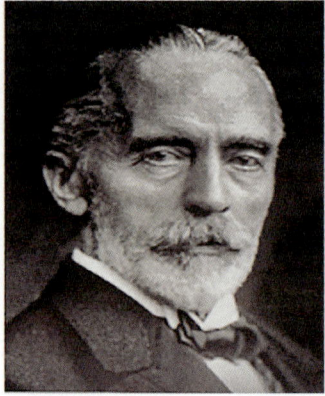
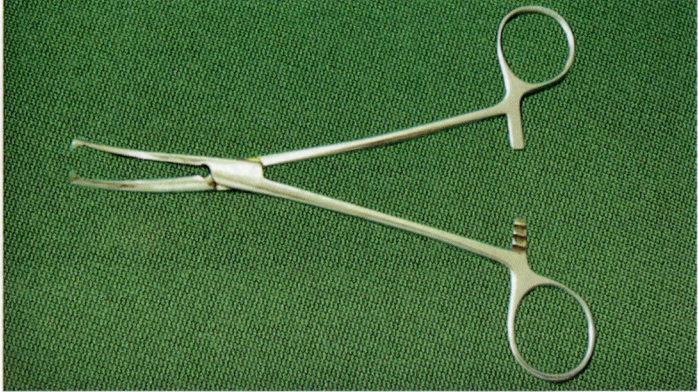

Emil Theodor Kocher (1841–1917)

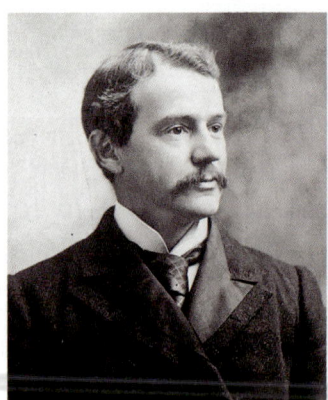
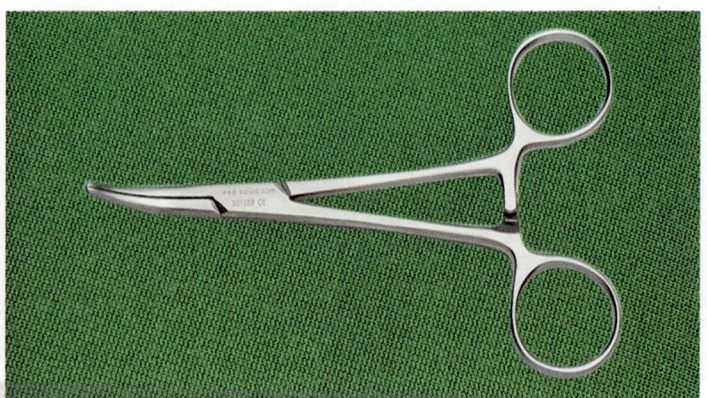

Howard Atwood Kelly (1858–1943)

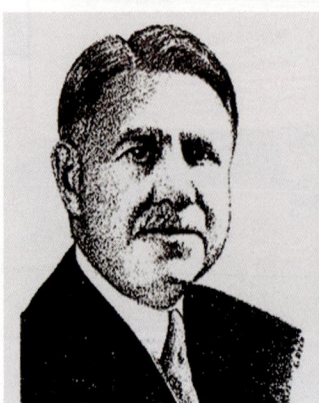
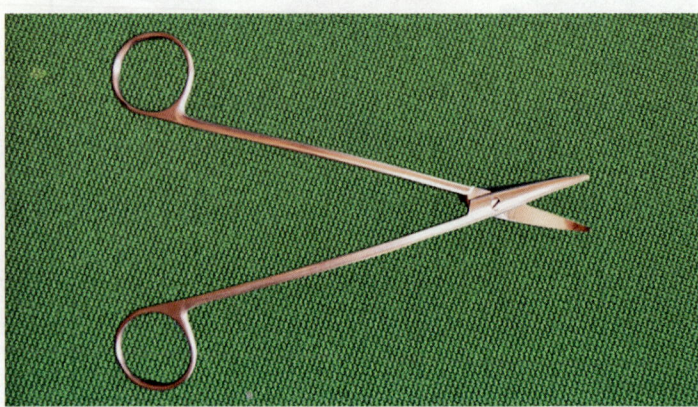

Myron Firth Metzenbaum (1876–1944)

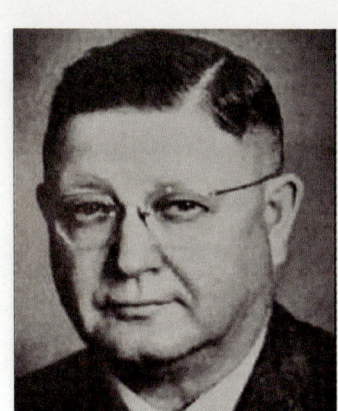
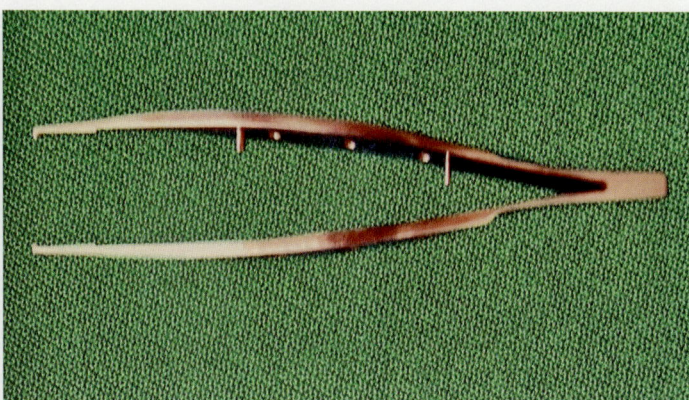

Alfred W Adson (1887–1951)

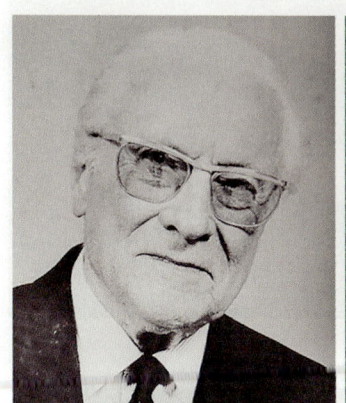
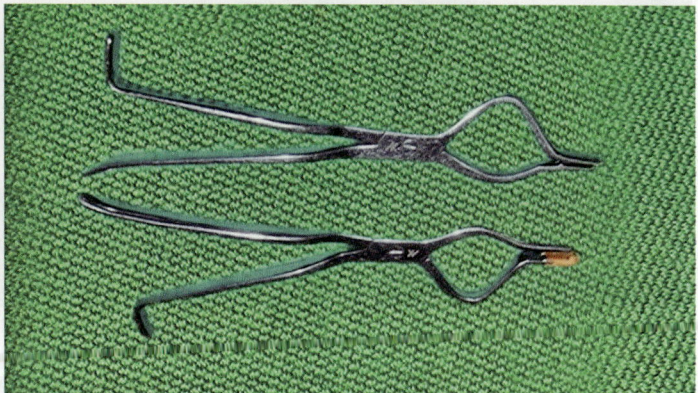

NL Rowe

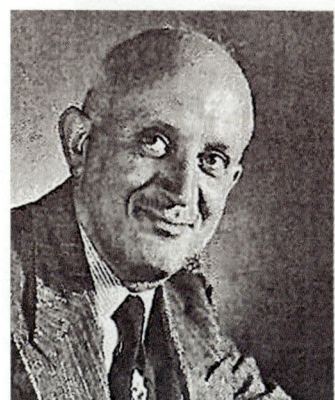
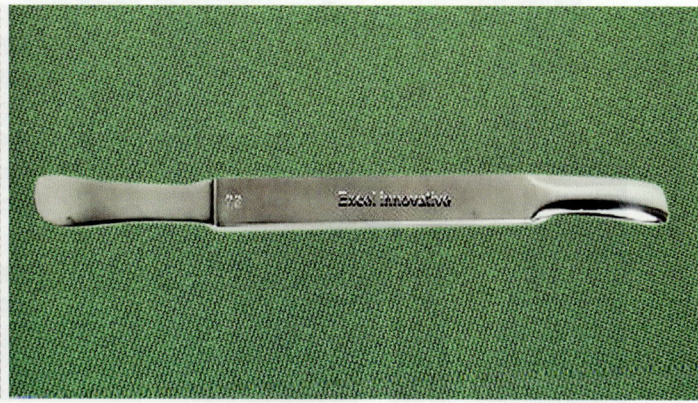

Harry M Seldin (1895–1975)

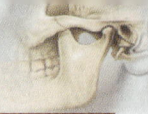

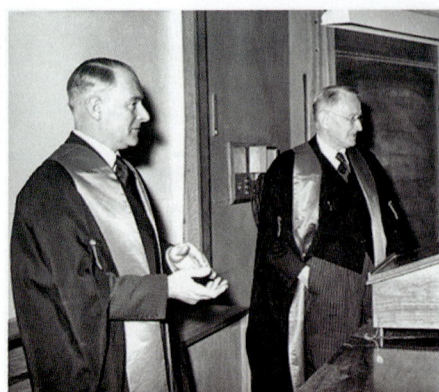

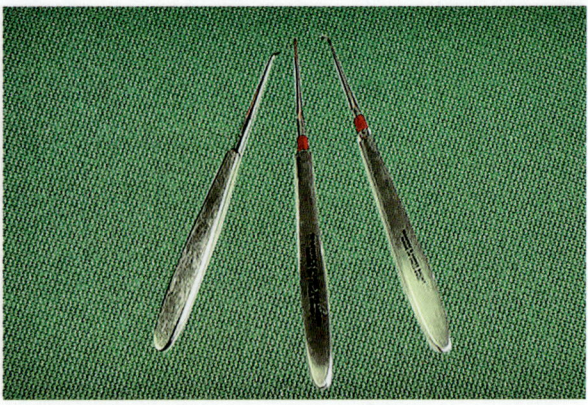

William Warwick James

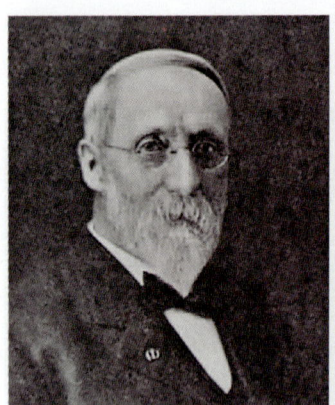

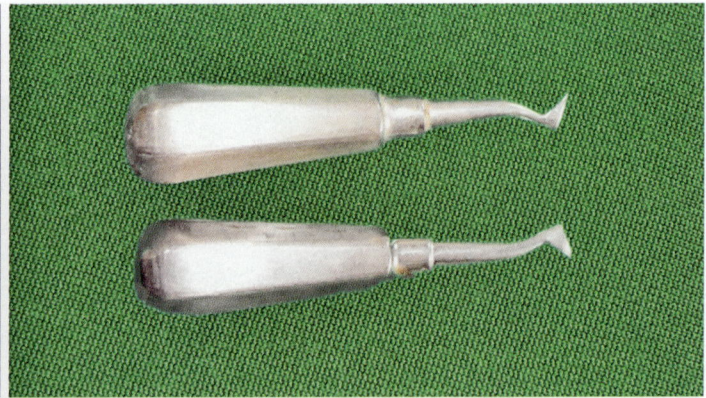

Matthew Henry Cryer (1840–1921)

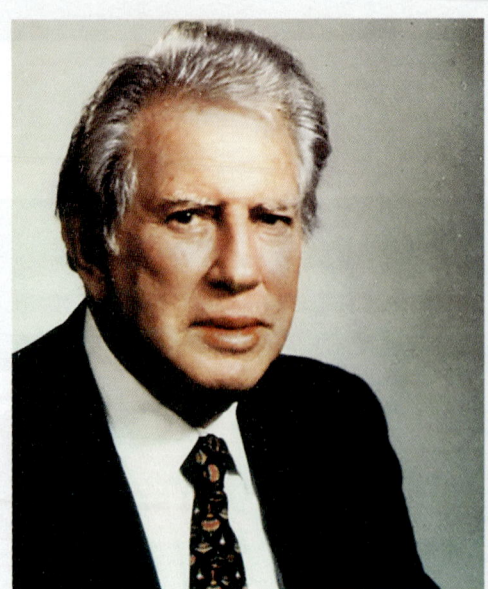

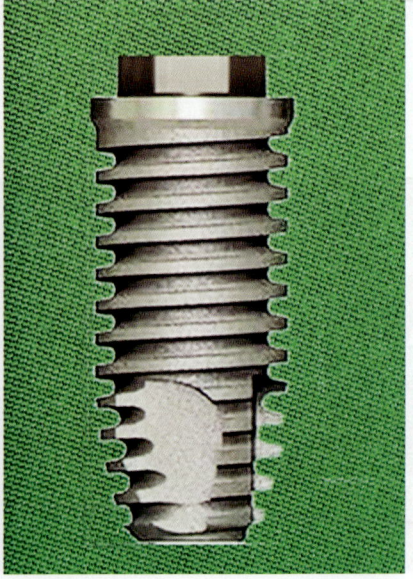

Dr Leonard I Linkow

Classification of Oral and Maxillofacial Surgical Instruments

Rahul Lature, Priyanka Tapsale, Fatima K Shaikh

A. GENERAL SURGICAL INSTRUMENTS CAN BE CLASSIFIED AS FOLLOWS

- Cutting instruments
- Grasping or holding instruments
- Haemostatic forceps
- Retractors
- Clamps and distractors
- Miscellaneous

B. EXODONTIA AND MINOR ORAL SURGICAL INSTRUMENTS CAN BE CLASSIFIED AS FOLLOWS

Exodontia Instruments Can be Classified as Follows

1. Forceps

- Maxillary anterior forceps
- Maxillary premolar forceps
- Maxillary molar forceps
- Maxillary cowhorn forceps
- Bayonet forceps or root forceps
- Maxillary 3rd molar forceps
- Mandibular anterior forceps
- Mandibular premolar forceps
- Mandibular molar forceps
- Mandibular cowhorn forceps
- Mandibular 3rd molar forceps

2. Elevators

- Straight elevators
  - Coupland elevator
  - London hospital pattern
- Angular elevators
  - Apexo elevator
  - Cryer's elevator
    - Crossbar pattern
    - Straight pattern

3. *Minor Oral Surgical Instruments Can be Classified as Follows*

- Diagnostic instruments
  - Mouth mirror
  - Straight probe
  - Explorer
  - Tweezers

- Cutting
  - Scalpel
  - Chisel
  - Mallet
  - Surgical burs
  - Surgical hand-piece

- Elevators and retractors
  - Right angled moon's retractor
  - No. 9 Molt periosteal elevator
  - Howarth's periosteal elevator
  - Austin retractor
  - Minnesota retractor
  - Cheek retractor

- Mouth gags
  - Mouth prop
  - Heister's mouth opener
  - Doyen's mouth gag
  - Fergusson's mouth gag

- Irrigation and debridement
  - Steel bowl
  - Bone curettes
  - Volkmann's scoop
  - Suction cannula
  - Syringes for irrigation

- Trimming and finishing
  - Bone ronguers
  - Miller's bone file

- Haemostat
  - Straight mosquito forceps
  - Curved mosquito forceps
  - Straight artery forceps
  - Curved artery forceps

- Suturing insrtuments
  - Dean's suture cutting scissors
  - Needle holder
  - Tissue forceps

C. MAXILLOFACIAL TRAUMA INSTRUMENTS CAN BE CLASSIFIED AS FOLLOWS

- Instruments for incision
  - Scalpel
  - Cautery
    - Unipolar
    - Bipolar
  - Laser system

- Instruments for dissection
  - Dissecting scissors
  - Mosquito forceps
  - Skin hook

- Instruments for reflection
  - Periosteal elevator
  - Periosteal stripper
  - Howarth's elevator

- Instruments for retraction
- Self-retaining retractors
  - Self-retaining mastoid retractor
  - Self-retaining skin retractor

- Plain hand held retractors
  - Orbital floor retractor
  - Langenback retractor
  - Obwegessor's ramus retractors
  - Condyle retractor
  - Chin retractor
  - Channel retractor
  - Mandibular body retractor
  - Sigmoid notch retractor
  - Doyen's raspatory (Rib retractor)
  - Tongue Depressor
  - Weider tongue retractor
  - 'C' shaped retractor (Deaver's retractor)
  - Universal retractor
  - Nerve hook (Dandy nerve hook)

- Instruments for curettage
  - Soft tissue curettes

- Instruments for reduction
  - Rowe's bone holding forceps
  - Bone reduction forceps
  - Kocher's toothed heavy artery forceps
  - Rowe's maxillary disimpaction forceps
  - Hayton William's forceps
  - Asch's nasal septal forceps

- Walsham septum straightening forceps
- Bristow's zygoma elevator
- Rowe's modification of Bristow's zygoma elevator
- Zygoma hook (Poswillo's pattern)
- Bone awl (Kelseyfry's bone awl)

- Instruments for osteotomy
  - Gigli's wire saw and introducer
  - Osteotome
  - Bone cutter
  - Rib shear
  - Bone gouge

- Instruments for intermaxillary fixation
  - Wire twister
  - Wire cutter
  - Erich's arch bar

- Instruments for internal fixation
  - Titanium screws
  - Titanium plates
  - Self-retaining screw driver
  - Screw driver
  - Plate cutters (paired)
  - Plate bending pliers
  - Mini plate holder
  - Plate introducing forceps
  - Erich's arch bar
  - Transbuccal trocar system

- Instruments for closure
  - Surgical needle
  - Needle holder
  - Adson's tissue forceps
  - Dean's suture cutting scissors

D. DISTRACTION OSTEOGENESIS DEVICES CAN BE CLASSIFIED AS FOLLOWS

- Extraoral distractors
  - External mandibular distractor—unidirectional
  - External mandibular distractor—bidirectional
  - External midface distractor

- Intraoral distractors
  - Intraoral alveolar ridge distractor
  - Intraoral ramus distractor
  - Intraoral distractor for mandible
  - Intraoral distractor for maxilla

- Instruments for adapting, fixing and activating the distractors

  - *For activating*
    - Plate holding forceps
    - Modelling pliers
    - Activator measuring devices
    - Activation arm disconnecting forceps
    - Screw driver

  - *For fixing*
    - Schanz screws
    - Plate cutters
    - Mini implants screws

E. ADVANCED INSTRUMENTS CAN BE CLASSIFIED AS FOLLOWS

- Instruments for exodontia
  - Physics forceps
  - Powered periotomes

- Instruments for incisions and closure
  - Lasers
  - Skin staples

- Instruments used for minimally invasive surgical techniques
  - Endoscopic instruments
  - Piezosurgery unit
  - Robotics for surgery

Sterilization of Surgical Instruments

Deepak Motwani, Kiran Raddar, Kartiken, Gopal Nagargoje

Sterilization is defined as removal or inactivation of all vegetative pathogenic and non-pathogenic micro-organisms along with all spore forms.

Centre for Disease Control has classified instruments according to degree of risk of transmission of infections. It was put forth by Spaulding. Classified into three categories—critical, semi-critical, non-critical.

- **Critical Instruments:** Instruments which penetrate the human body tissues and cavities and get contaminated with micro-organisms. These are sterilized by high level sterilization.

  Example: Scalpel, chisels, ronguers, burs, files, scalers.

- **Semi-critical Instruments:** Instruments which contact mucous membranes, non-intact skin surfaces. These require intermediate level sterilization.

  Example: Flexible orthoscope, endoscope.

- **Non-critical Instruments:** These come in contact with only intact skin surfaces, mucous membranes. These are sterilized by low level disinfection.

  Example: Blood pressure cuff, pulse oximeter.

Stages of Sterilization are as follows

- Presoaking
- Cleaning
- Corrosion control or lubrication
- Packaging
- Sterilization
- Handling sterile instruments
- Storage
- Distribution

Various Agents used in Sterilization are as follows

- **Physical agents:**
  - Sunlight
  - Dry heat
  - Drying
  - Moist heat
  - Boiling

- Radiation
- Ultrasonic and sonic vibrations
- Filtration

- **Chemical agents**
  - Alcohols like ethyl alcohol
  - Aldehydes like formaldehyde
  - Dyes
  - Halogens
  - Phenols
  - Surface active agents
  - Metallic salts
  - Gases like ethylene oxide

Four Widely Accepted Methods of Sterilization are

- Steam under pressure, viz. autoclave.
- Chemical vapour pressure sterilization—chemiclave.
- Dry heat sterilization—dryclave.
- Ethylene oxide sterilization.

Amongst these four, autoclave is the most widely used method of sterilizing and has been explained in detail as follows.

Autoclave

The name 'Autoclave' comes from the Greek word *autos* meaning "self", and Latin word *clavis* meaning "key". It was invented by Charles Chamberland in 1879. An autoclave is an unit which uses high pressure at high temperature and steam for sterilization of instruments.

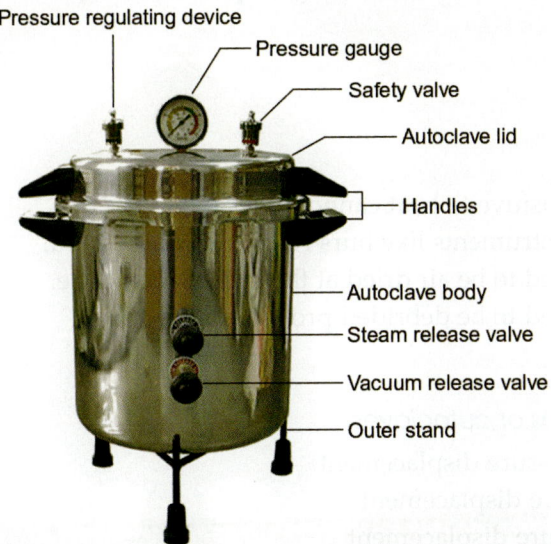

Top loading autoclave

For medical and dental uses, following combinations of temperature and holding time can be used:

Method	Temperature (degree C)	Holding time (in minutes)	Pressure
Autoclave	121	15	15 Psi
	126	10	20 Psi
	134	3	30 Psi

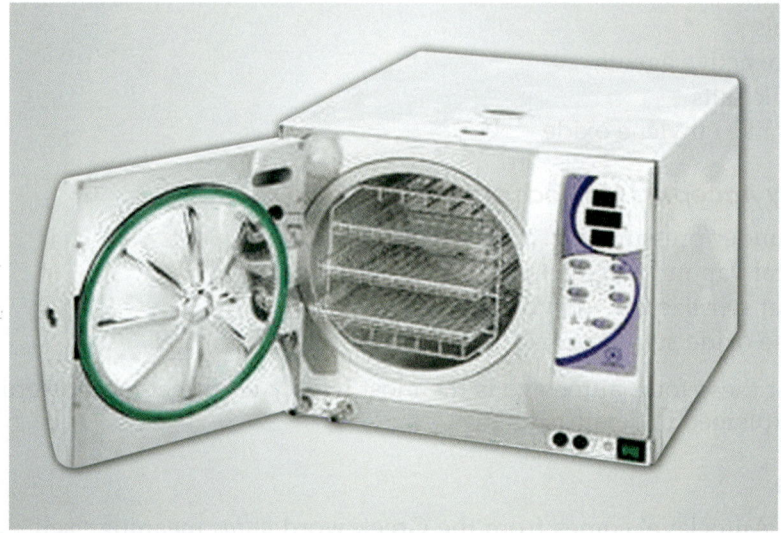

Front loading autoclave

Advantages

- Most rapid method of sterilization
- Most effective method for cloth surgical packs, towel packs, etc.
- Dependable
- Economical
- Verifiable

Disadvantages

- Instruments sensitive to heat cannot be used.
- Carbon steel instruments like burs rust when autoclaved.
- Instruments need to be air dried at the end of each cycle.
- Instruments need to be debrided properly before use.

Types of Autoclave

There are four types of autoclaves:

- Downward pressure displacement
- Positive pressure displacement
- Negative pressure displacement
- Triple vacuum autoclave

- **Downward pressure displacement:** It is so called because of its method of air removal in the sterilization chamber. Also called 'gravity displacement unit'.
- **Positive pressure displacement:** Steam is created in a separate chamber and held there until the proper amount to displace all the air in the sterilization chamber. Steam is then released in the sterilization chamber. Functionally, this one is better than previously mentioned autoclave.
- **Negative pressure displacement:** This is one of the most accurate types of autoclaves available.
  Once sterilization chamber door is closed, a vacuum pump removes the air. Steam is created in a second, separate chamber. Once the air has been completely removed from the sterilization chamber, the steam is then released into it in a pressure blast. It is able to achieve a high "sterility assurance level" but the system can be quite large and costly.
- **Triple vacuum autoclave:** It is similar to negative pressure displacement autoclave. The autoclaving cycle is repeated thrice.
  It is suitable for all types of instruments.

Sterilization Control

The quality of sterilization achieved in an autoclave can be checked by various methods, broadly divided into:

- **Biological indicators:** *Bacillus stearothermophilus* spores are used as the test organism at 121°C for 15 minutes as they get killed at about its 12th minute. 10^6 spores are used on the test strip and then incubated at 55°C for 5 days. *Geobacillus stearothermophilus* is also used, wherein a pH sensitive strip is used and shows change in colour at appropriate temperature.
- **Chemical indicators:** Halochromic chemical compounds like carboxylic acids, amines, etc. show different colors at different pH. These are used to check quality of sterility.

  Autoclave tape: It changes colour due to heat and steam at 134°C. However, it does not indicate complete sterility.
- **Alloy indicators:** Some alloys melt when a desired temperature is reached. These are used to check quality of sterilization by the means of the temperature reached.

  Example: Titanium alloy screws.
- **Computer controlled indicators:** Computer controlled—F_0 (F naught) value is also used to check for quality of sterilization cycle. These values are set for number of minutes of sterilization equivalent to 121°C (250°F) at 100 kPa (15 psi) above atmospheric pressure for 15 minutes.

General Surgery Instruments

Hanumant T Karad, Sanjay S Byakode, Ahtesham Ahmad

CUTTING INSTRUMENTS

DISSECTING SCISSORS

This is also called Mayo's scissors and is popularly called tissue scissors.

Indication

- This is used to dissect tissue planes during surgical operations and to cut or divide important structures.

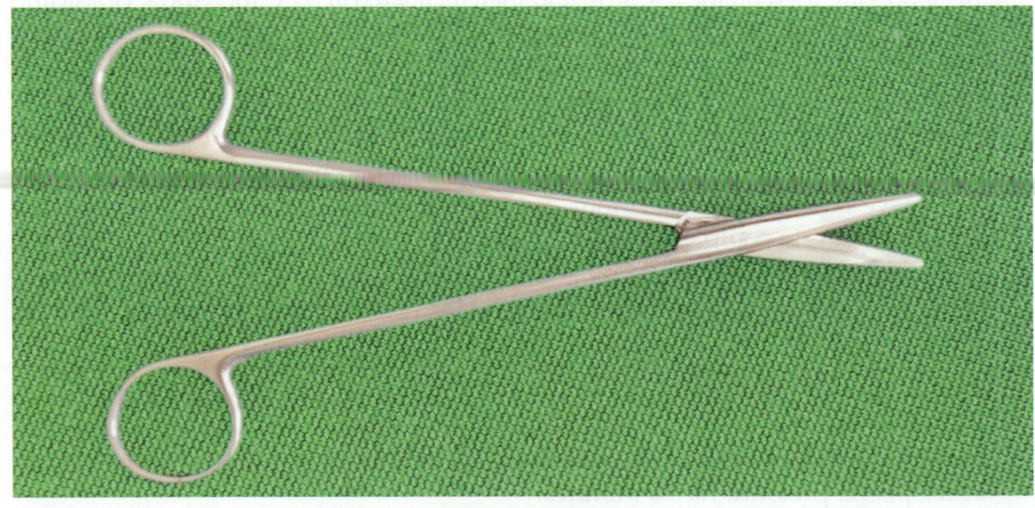

Dissecting scissors

HUMBY'S KNIFE

This instrument has a handle and long sheath. There is a screw at the operating end, with which prior adjustments should be done.

Indication

- The instrument is used to harvest skin grafts. Hence, it is also called skin grafting knife.

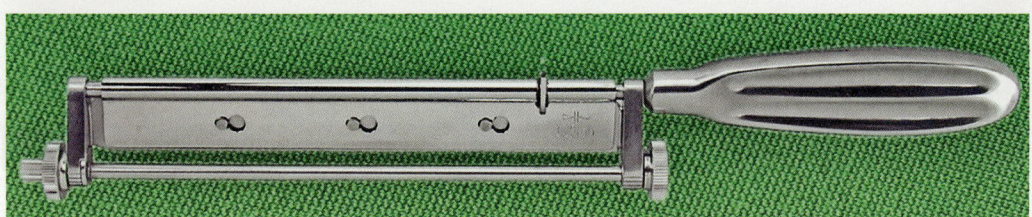

Humby's knife

KOCHER'S THYROID DISSECTOR

This has long handles and the operating end is small and blunt with an opening. A few longitudinal serrations are present at the tip.

Indications

- This is used to dissect the upper pole of the thyroid gland.
- This instrument can also be used to dissect the isthmus of the thyroid gland from the trachea.
- Silk thread can be fed into the opening so as to ligate the vascular pedicle or isthmus.

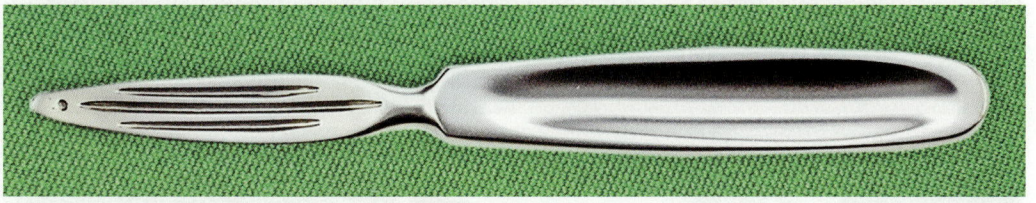

Kocher's thyroid dissector

SUTURE CUTTING SCISSORS (DEAN'S)

It can be straight or curved and angulated or non-angulated.

Angulation at the joint or at tip facilitates access to the posterior area of the oral cavity. It has long delicate handles and short cutting edges.

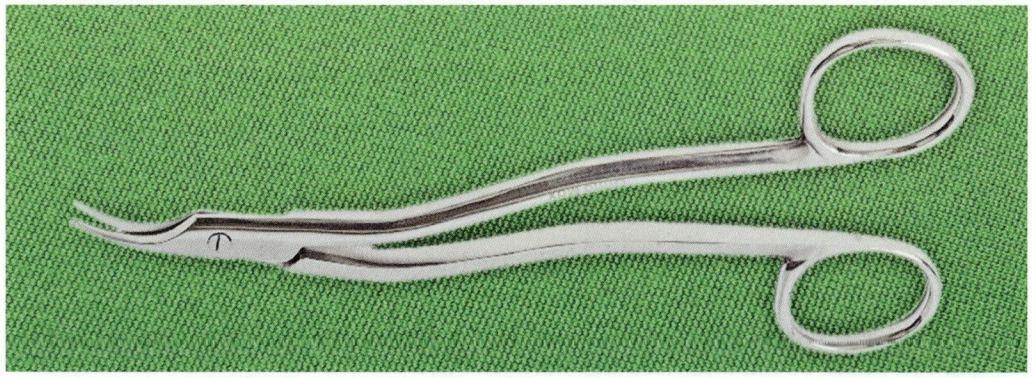

Suture cutting scissors (Dean's)

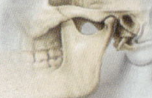

Indication

- It is used to cut the sutures or knots.

GRASPING OR HOLDING FORCEPS

ALLIS TISSUE HOLDING FORCEPS

The forceps with locking handle and blades have delicate teeth.

It has a ratchet and triangular expansion at the tip, where serrations are present and handle is longer than beaks.

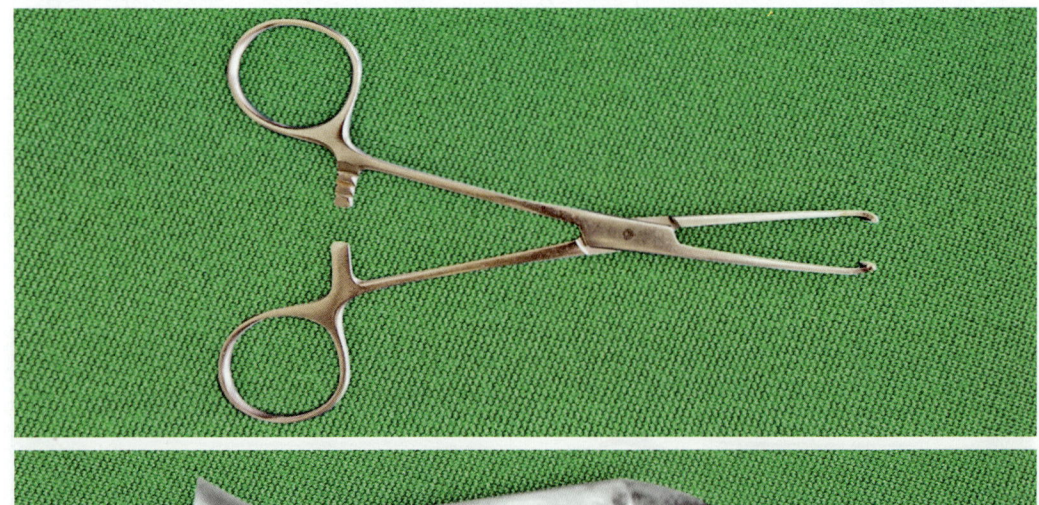

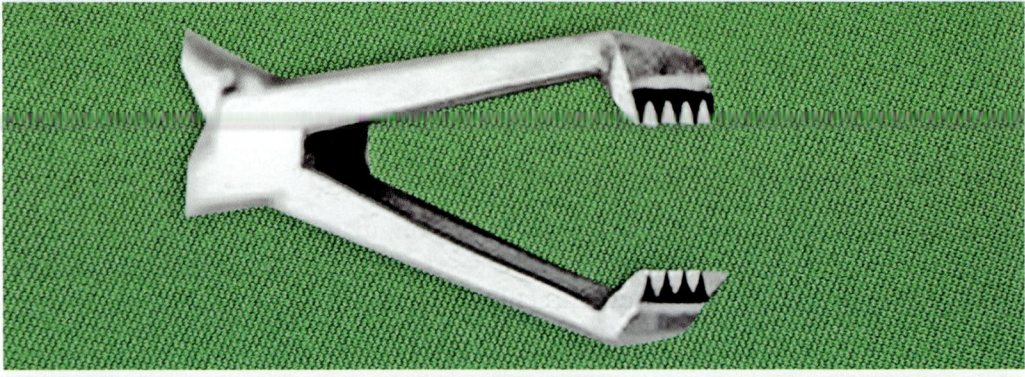

Allis tissue holding forceps

Precautions

- They are never used on soft tissues or on tissues which have to be left in the mouth as it results in a large amount of tissue destruction due to crushing.

Indications

- It can be used to hold tough structures such as fascia and aponeurosis, etc.
- To provide tension during tissue dissection.
- To hold and retract the tissues (generally for tissues that will be excised).
- Should never be used to hold the skin directly.
- Held in the same way as needle holder.

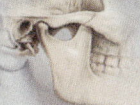

ADSON DISSECTING TISSUE FORCEPS

Delicate forceps, their tip forms a 'w' shape when held in a closed position.

They are so designed that the tissues experience minimum trauma during the surgery.

They are often referred to as the rat tooth forceps.

Two Types

- Plain/non-toothed—(no tooth at the tips) have serrations on the inner aspect of the tip to aid in grip, used to hold delicate structures like delicate muscles, fascia and facial skin, blood vessels or nerves.

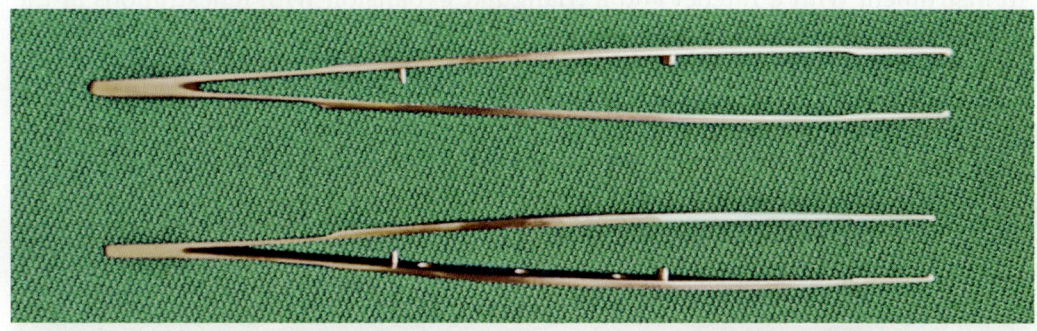

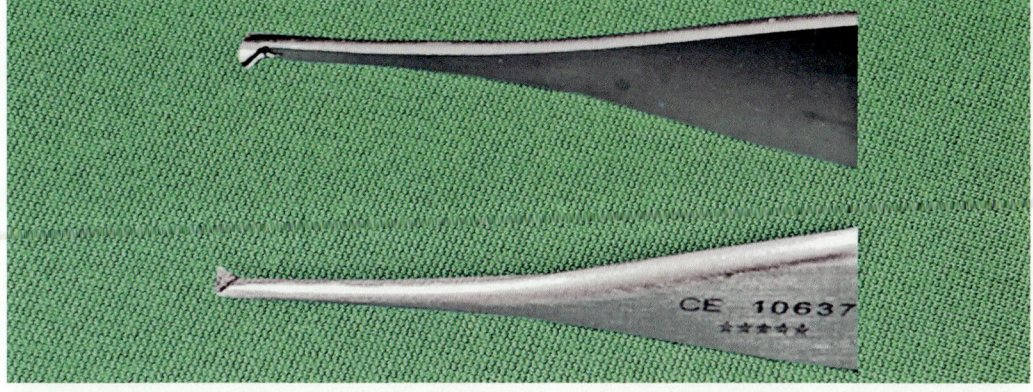

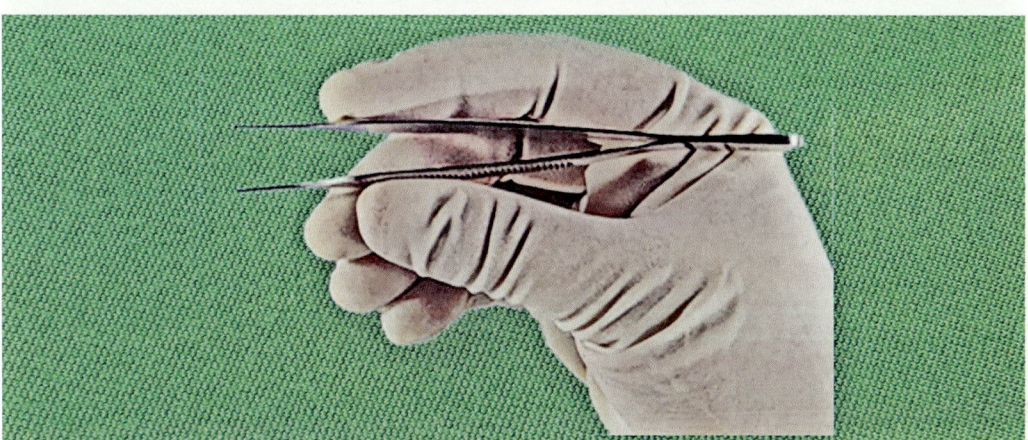

Adson dissecting tissue forceps

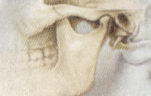

- Toothed—(having teeth at the tips) used to hold tough structures like skin, coarse muscle and fascia.
- They are of different lengths, i.e. 4/6/8 inches, and are used according to the need.
- Microadson forceps (used for precise and fine handling of the soft tissue).
- Always held in pen grip.

Indication

The forceps are very useful to 'pick' individual layers such as mucosa and submucosa during anastomosis.

BABCOCK'S FORCEPS

An instrument with a ratchet and a triangular expansion with fenestrations at the operating end. It does not have any teeth.

    More delicate and less traumatic than Allis' forceps.

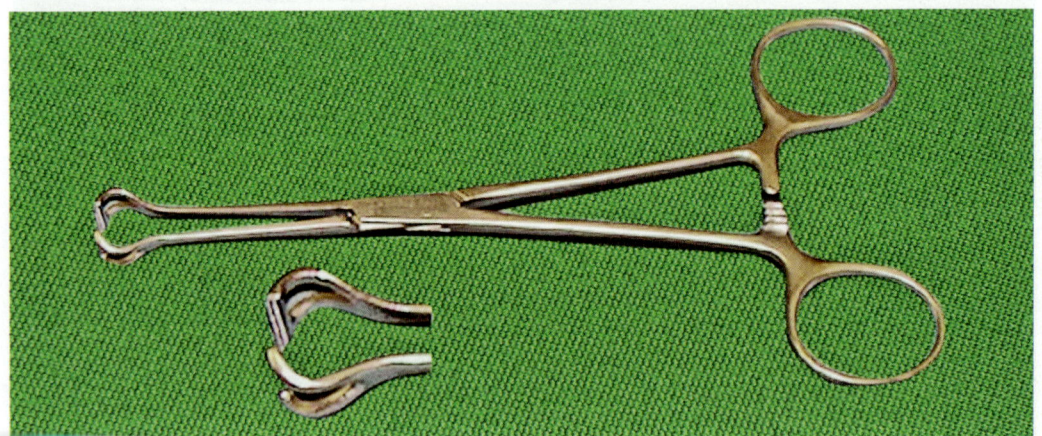

Babcock's forceps

Indication

- Used to hold enlarged lymph nodes or any glandular tissue.

    For example, intestine, thyroid gland, mesoappendix, uterine tubes, etc.

CHEATLE'S FORCEPS

It is a long instrument having a curved shaft. The handle has no lock.

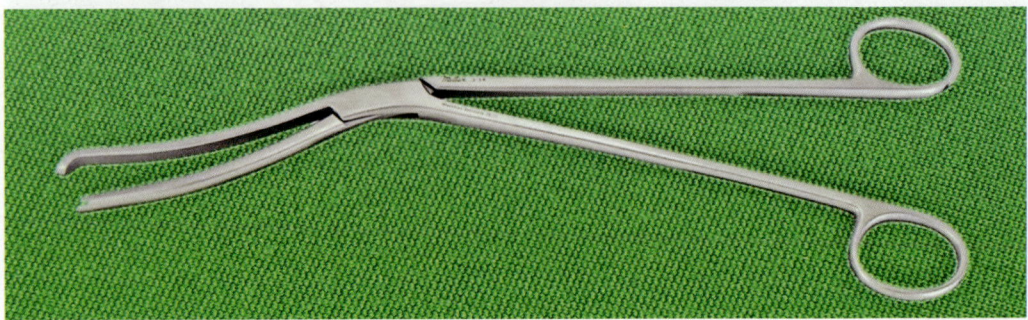

Cheatle's forceps

Indication

- Used for picking up sterile instruments from trays and linens from the drum. Stored in a container containing antiseptic solution.

KOCHER'S FORCEPS

This is similar to an artery forceps with serrations.
It is available as curved and straight.
There is a sharp tooth at the tip of the instrument, hence it has a better grip.

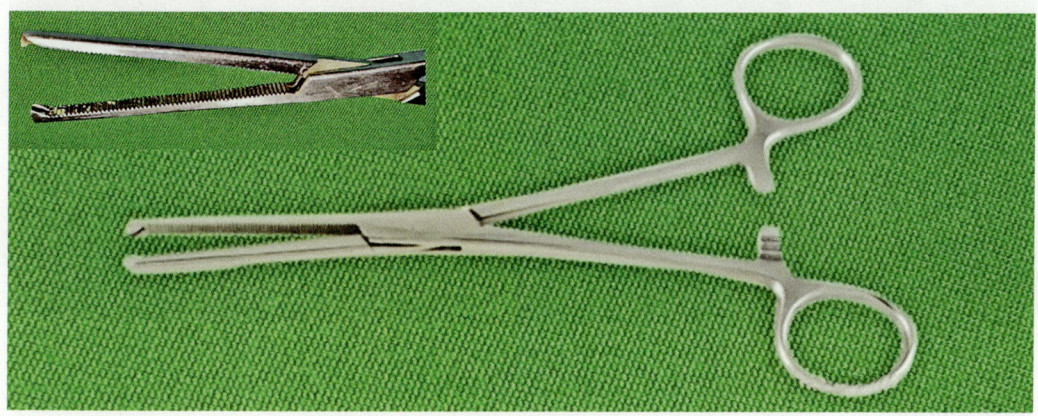

Kocher's forceps

Indications

- Used to hold tough structures such as aponeurosis, fascia, and muscles.
- During thyroidectomy, it can be used to hold the strap muscles for dividing them.
- To hold rib during rib resection.

LANE'S FORCEPS

This is similar to babcock's forceps, but the tip is more broad, expanded with a bigger opening.

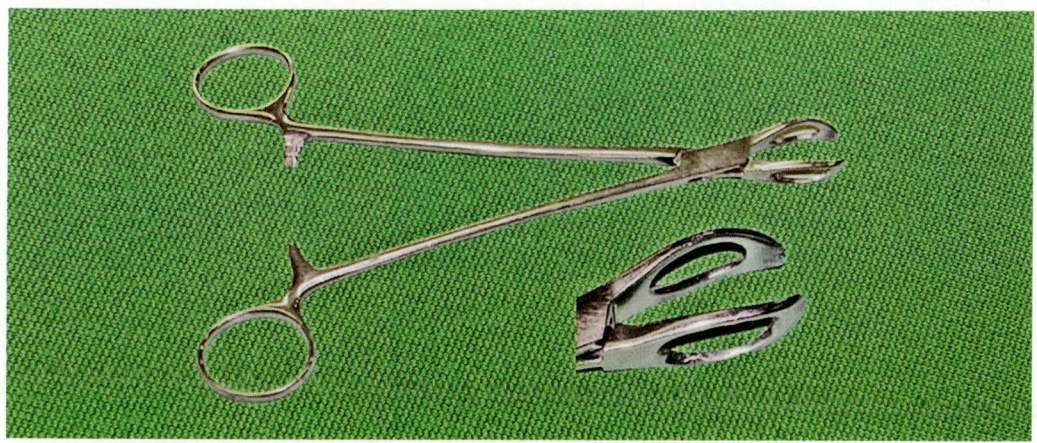

Lane's forceps

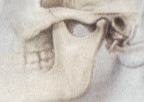

Indication

- It is used to hold appendix.

LISTER'S SINUS FORCEPS

This is like an artery forceps which has no ratchet. Serrations are confined to the tip so as to hold the wall of an abscess cavity. Straight, long and slender instrument with narrow blades. The tip is rounded and bulbous.

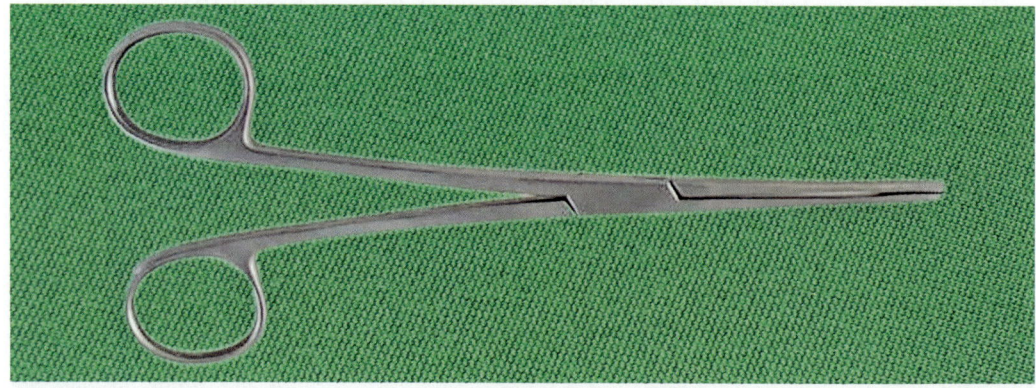

Lister's sinus forceps

Indications

- To open an abscess by Hilton's method to break the locule.
- To hold a small piece of gauze between the blades to clean a cavity.
- To dissect out sinus and/or fistulous tract.

NEEDLE HOLDER

This is a long instrument with a ratchet at the non-operating end. The operating end has two small blades with serrations.

Indications

- The instrument is used to hold the curved needle, which is used to suture the parts.
- A firm grip is essential to apply proper sutures.

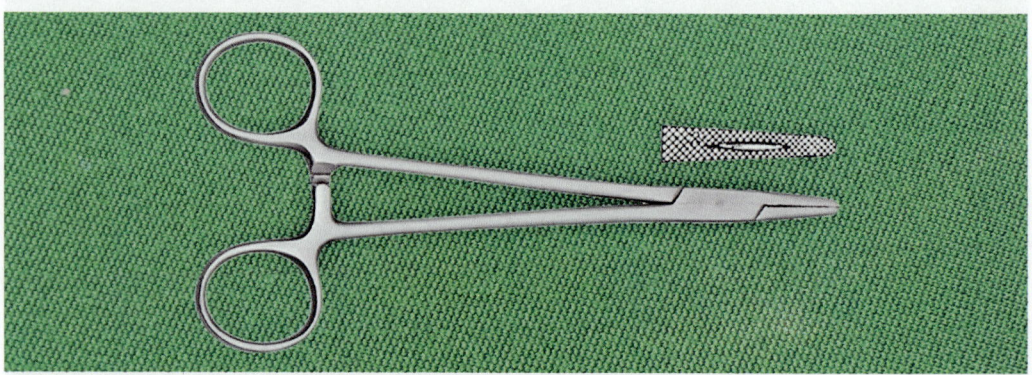

Needle holder

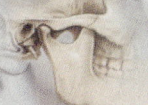
SKIN HOOK

It may have one or two very thin curved hooks at the end of the tool. The prongs of the skin hook instrument can be customized to the procedure performed. Some types of this surgical equipment have hooks that are very sharp and thin.

Other skin hooks feature prongs that are thick and have a dull tip.

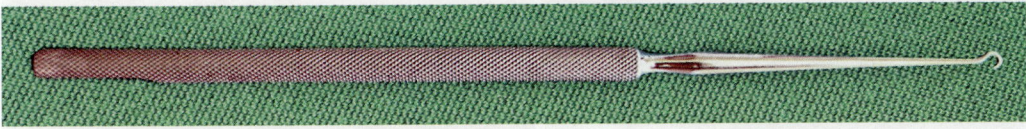

Skin hook

Indications

- A skin hook is a small instrument that is used to grasp, hold, and position delicate soft tissue during the suturing phase of surgical procedure.
- Skin hooks are used in many different medical procedures that require the gentle maneuvering of skin and soft tissue, including corrective surgical procedure on the eyes, suturing facial skin, and stitching the delicate individual layers of the skin.

SWAB HOLDING FORCEPS

This has a ratchet and two long blades. An instrument with long blades, expanded at the ends forming an oblong tip with central fenestration and transverse serrations.

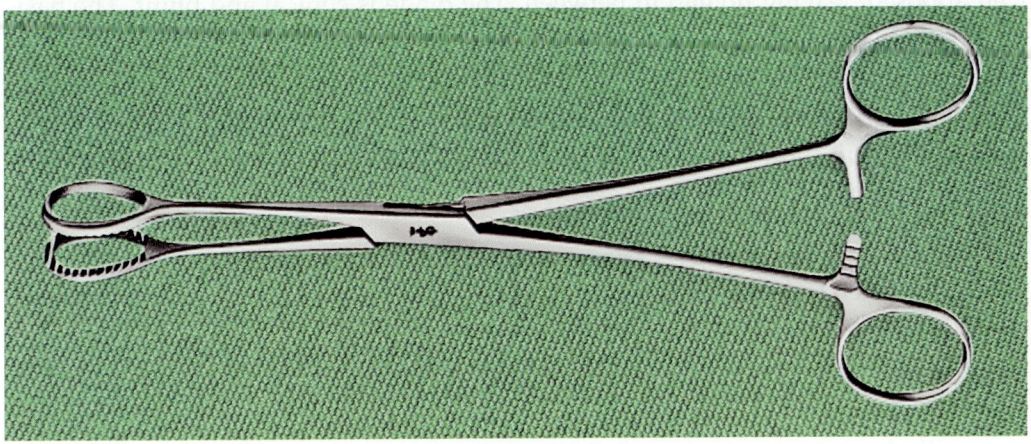

Swab holding forceps

Indications

- To hold a swab and clean the area of operation with an antiseptic solution preoperatively. To swab the throat, when there are profuse secretions in an unconscious patient.
- To hold the tongue and give anterior traction and, thus, preventing tongue fall and airway obstruction.

TRANSFER FORCEPS

- Heavy right angled forceps with heavy jaw.

Indication

Heavy forceps used to move instruments from one sterile area to another.

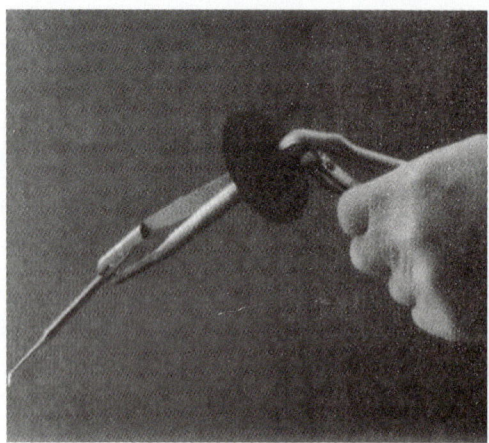
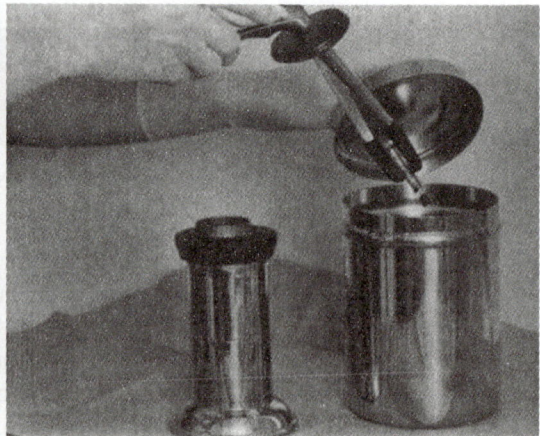

Transfer forceps

HAEMOSTATIC FORCEPS

ARTERY FORCEPS (HAEMOSTAT)

It is a light but strong instrument. These are hinged (locking) forceps having relatively long delicate beaks and unidirectional transverse serrations on the blades which are well apposed, leaving no gap in between. The blade is conical and blunt. The basic features of mosquito forcep are essentially the same as above except that these forceps are very small in size and has relatively pointed tips.

Classification on the Basis of Size and Shapes

- Small or mosquito, medium and large or pedicular.

Artery Forceps can also be Classified as

- Toothed type, e.g. Kocher's artery forceps, Lane's artery forceps.
- Non-toothed type, e.g. Crile's artery forceps, Spencer-well artery forceps, Halsted's artery forceps.

Indications

- They are used to control bleeding, not only from arteries, but also from veins and capillaries.
- Once the bleeding points are caught, they are coagulated or ligated. As tissue forceps for holding subcutaneous tissue and aponeurosis (but not skin or nerves).
- To drain an abscess by the Hilton's method. Straight artery, which is used to hold the stay sutures.
- To pick up necrotic tissue, granulation tissue, foreign bodies, tooth/root piece, small fragments of bone, etc.

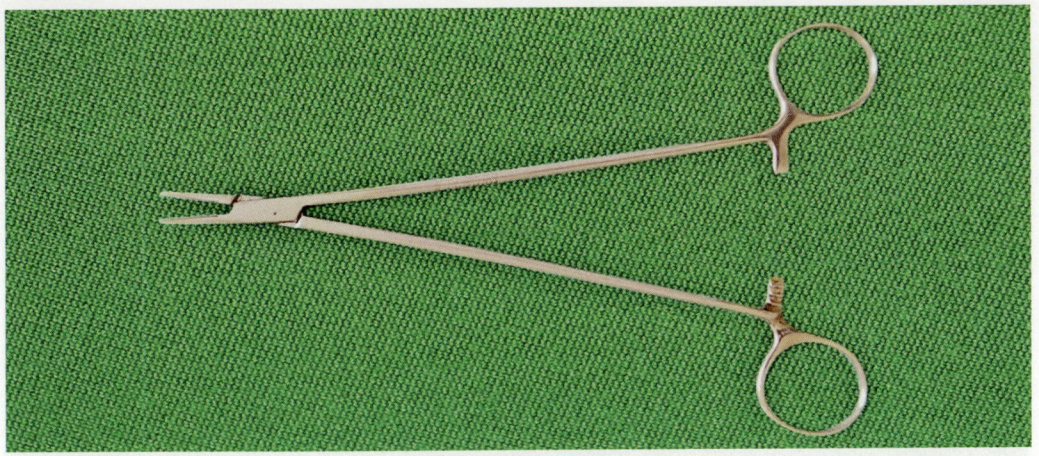

Straight artery forceps

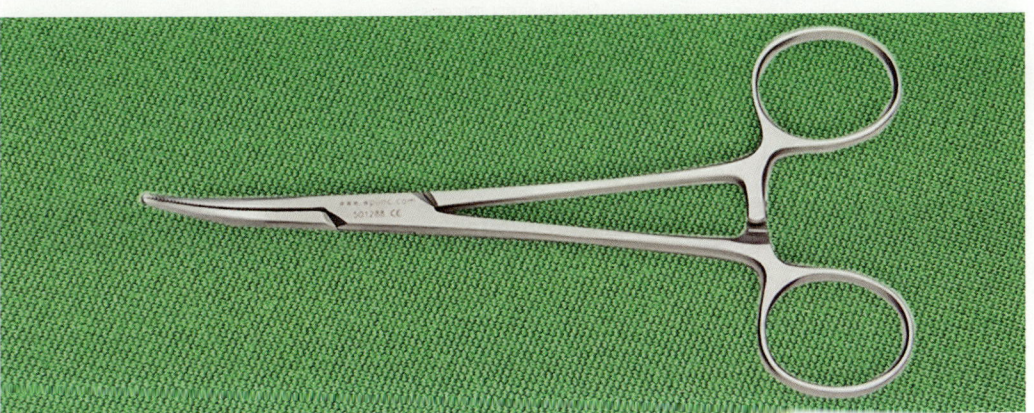

Curved artery forceps

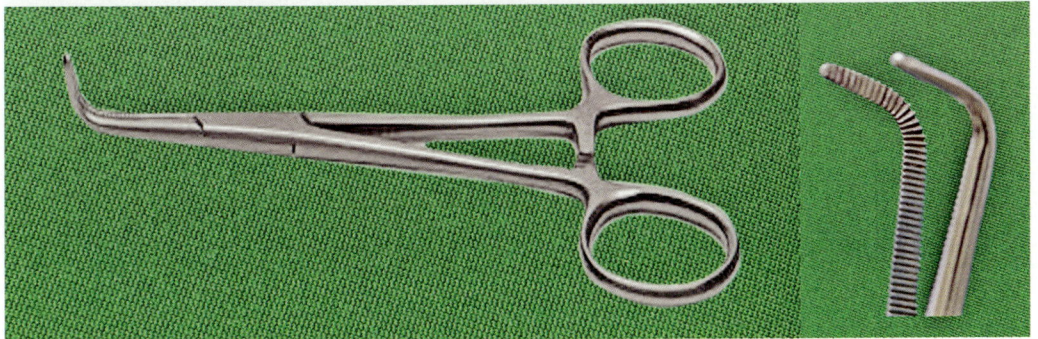

Mixter artery forceps

- Mixter forceps—useful for clamping vessels and separating tissue on vasculature that is deep within the body.
- Mosquito artery forceps for holding small pointed bleeding sites and to hold gauze-pellets for blunt dissection.

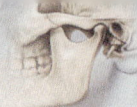

NEGU'S ARTERY FORCEPS

It is a stout, long jawed forceps. The jaws are bent in the form of a hook. The inner margins of the jaw are transversely serrated.

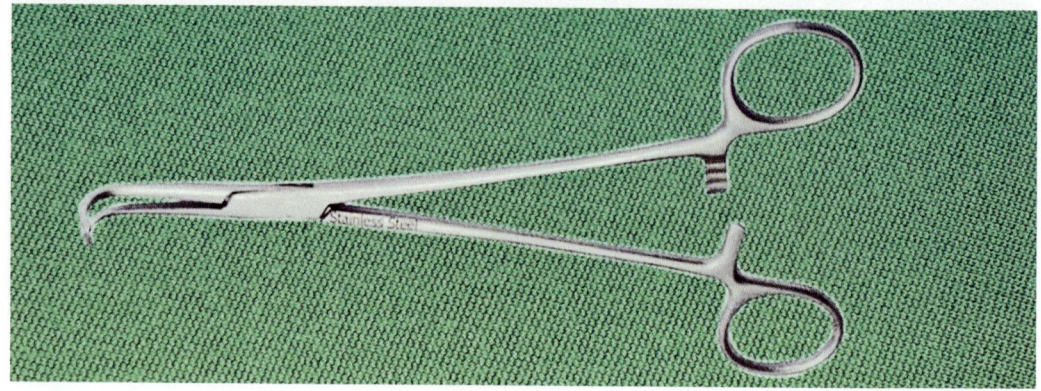

Negu's artery forceps

Indication

- It is used to ligate the vessels present at depth. The bleeder is held with a straight artery forceps and then Negu's curved artery forceps is used to ligate it.

RETRACTORS

CAT'S PAW RETRACTOR

Instrument resembles a cat's paw. Thin metallic double ended/single ended instrument. Blade has prongs that are curved at tip. Double ended/senn retractor with other end has a broad curved blade to retract small amount of soft tissue.

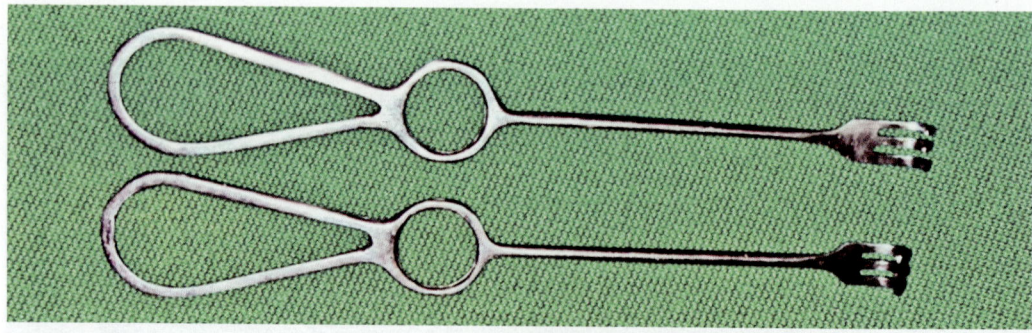

Cat's paw retractor

Precaution

- Care should be taken not to apply excessive force which might lead to soft tissue damage.

Indication

- It is used for retraction of a small amount of soft tissue.

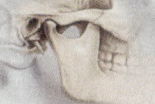

RIB SPREADER

This is a strong and heavy instrument having two long blades.

Indication

- Rib spreader is used once an incision is deepened through the intercostal spaces and the pleura is opened, and by rotating the latch handle the ribs are spread apart.

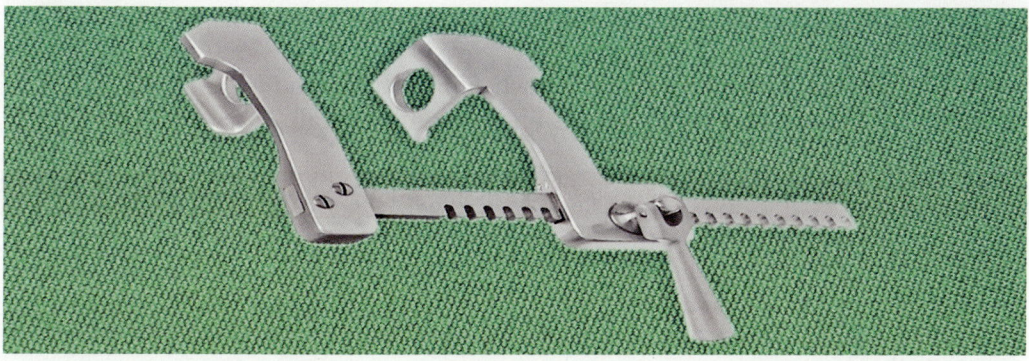

Rib spreader

LANGENBACK RETRACTOR

It has a long handle and L-shaped blade. Available in different sizes of handle and blade (width and length). It can be single/double ended.

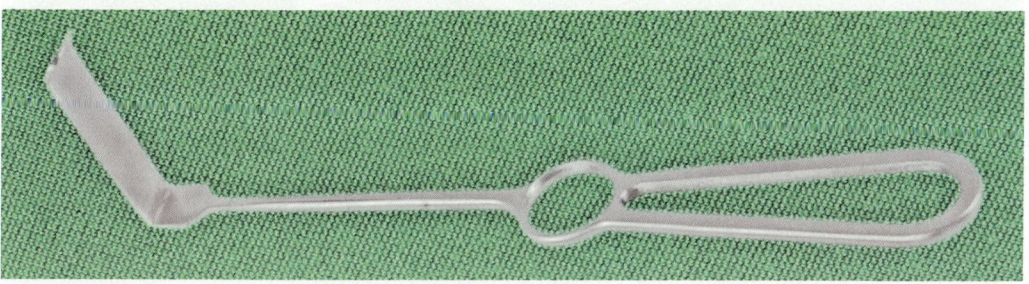

Langenback retractor

Common Types Are

- Standard (edge of the blade points towards the handle).
- Reverse (edge of the blade points away from the handle) edge of the blade can take support to retract tissues.

Indications

- To retract incised edges and soft tissue mass.
- To allow visualization of deeper tissues and to reduce fracture fragments (reverse type).

TONGUE DEPRESSOR

'L' shaped with broad, smooth blade to depress or retract the tongue.
Malleable tongue depressor

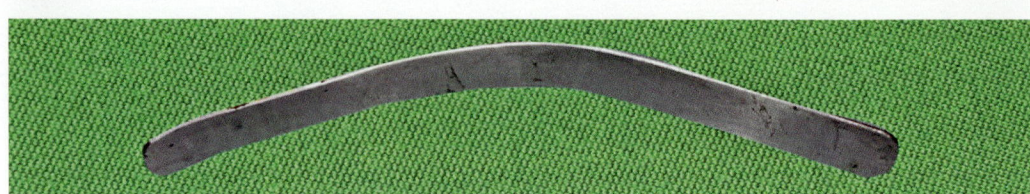

Tongue depressor

Indications

- To depress the tongue during endotracheal intubation and extubation.
- For inspection of oral cavity, tonsils and pharyngeal wall.

CLAMPS AND DISTRACTION

FORCEPS TYPE TOWEL CLIP

The beckhaus type towel clip has a box joint and it is like forceps. The tip of the instrument curves towards each other, pointed and overlaps each other which penetrate the drapes.

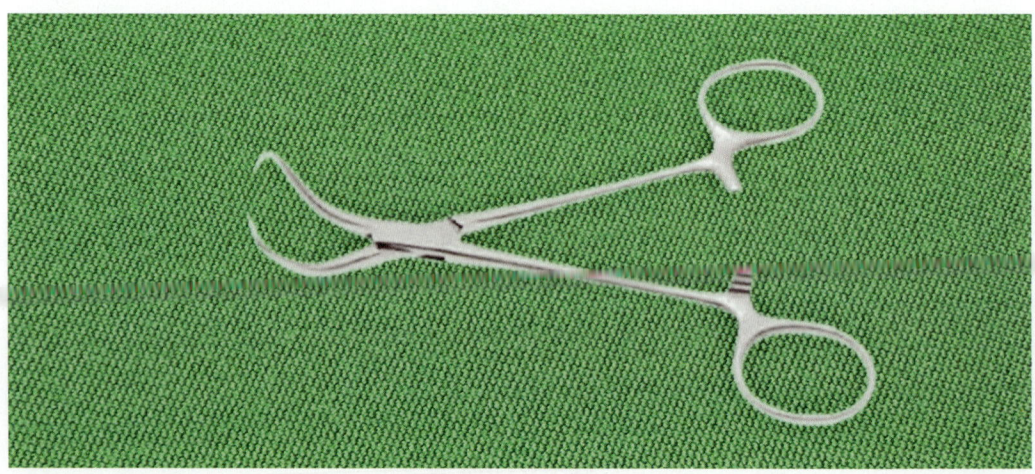

Forceps type towel clip

Indication

- Towel clips are used to maintain surgical towel and drape in correct position during an operation. To stabilize suction tubes, motor cables and other cables are used.

PINCHTER TYPE TOWEL CLIP

Jones type has spring joint. Tip of the instruments curves towards each other, pointed and overlaps each other which penetrate drapes.

Indication

- Towel clips are used to maintain surgical towels and drapes in correct position during an operation. To stabilize suction tubes, motor cables and other cables are used.

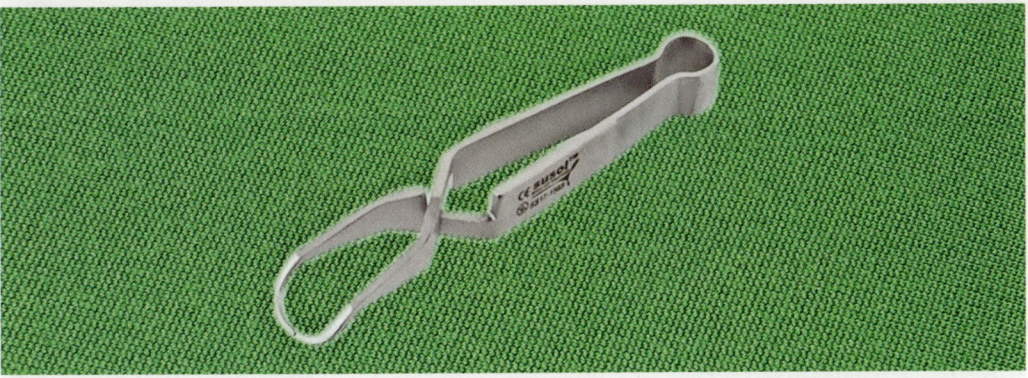

Pinchter type towel clip

MISCELLANEOUS

FOLEY'S SELF-RETAINING URINARY CATHETER

- This is made of latex with silicon coating.
- At tip there is a bulb and capacity of which, is written at the other end.
- Tip is blunt with 2–3 openings and balloon present.
- The other end has two tubes—the wider one for urine passage and the narrower one to inflate and deflate the balloon.

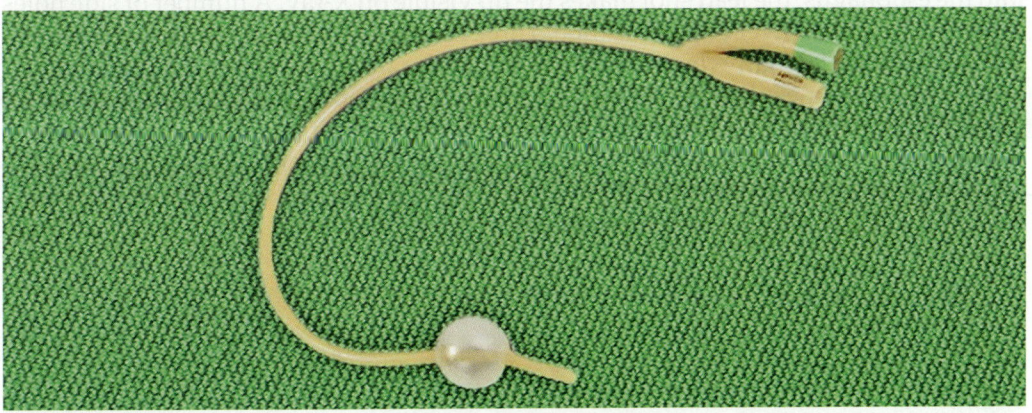

Foley's self-retaining urinary catheter

Procedure

- After introducing the catheter, the bulb is inflated using saline. Before inflating the bulb, one must make sure that the catheter is in the urinary bladder, not in the urethra. This is assessed by free flow of urine.
- After the usage, it is removed by deflating the bulb.

Indications

- To evacuate the bladder.
- It can also be used to drain the peritoneal cavity as in biliary peritonitis.

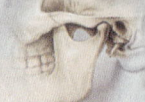

STEEL BOWL/GALLIPOT

A simple stainless steel bowl with variety of sizes, small and large, are available.

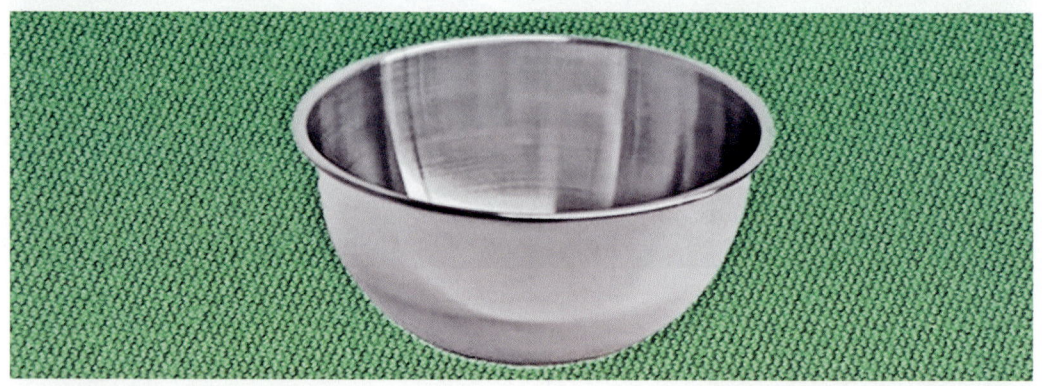

Steel bowl/gallipot

Indication

To keep gauze piece immersed in betadine solution.

RYLE'S TUBE/NASOGASTRIC TUBE

It is a meter long, rubber or synthetic transparent tube. At the end there are lead shots inside it with blunt tip. The lead shot at the tip facilitates the passing down of the tube into the esophagus, the lead shot makes the tip visible on X-ray. A number of side holes is present near the lower end of the tube. Three black circular marking are present over it, 1st marking at 40 cm which when present at the tip of the nose indicates that the lower end of the nasogastric tube is lying at gastro-esophageal junction in an adult patient. 2nd marking at 50 cm which when present at nasal tip indicates tip of the tube is in the body of the stomach and the 3rd marking at 60 cm which when presents at the nasal tip indicates that the tip of the tube is lying at the pylorus. Some tube also has a fourth marking at about 65 cm from the tip.

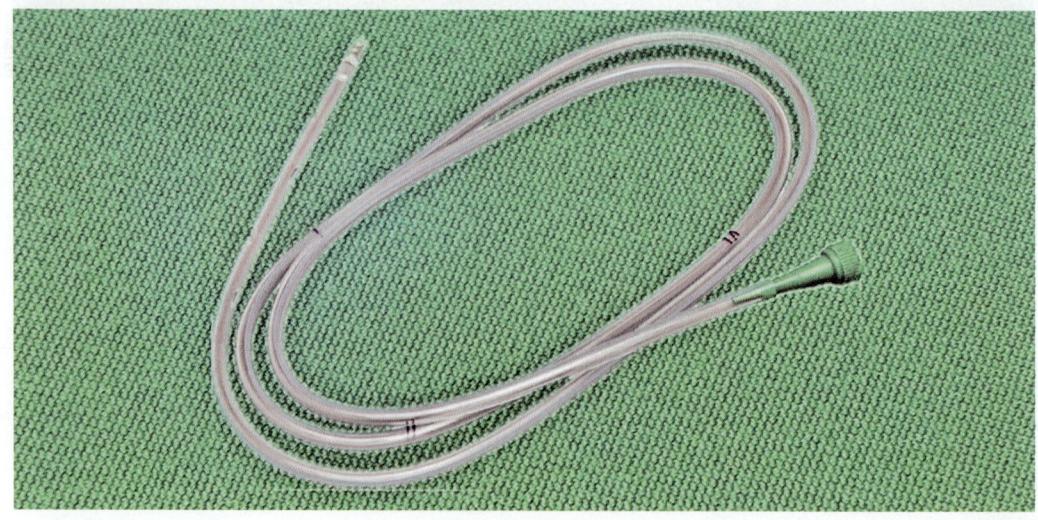

Ryle's tube/nasogastric tube

Procedure

i. A sterile tube is taken and the patient is explained about the procedure before inserting the tube.

ii. The patient is positioned either in a lying down position with extension of neck or is made to sit on the bed.

iii. The patient is asked to drink a glass of water.

iv. The tip of the tube is lubricated with liquid paraffin and is introduced through either of the two nostrils.

v. A local anaesthetic should not be used for lubrication as it abolishes the important protective mechanism, i.e. the cough reflex.

vi. The tube is pushed gently along the floor of the nose. Once the tube reaches the pharynx, there will be a tendency to cough or gag.

vii. At this moment reassure the patient and ask him to swallow the tube. The swallowing of tube can be facilitated by asking the patient to take sips of water from the glass given to him.

viii. Once the nasogastric tube has been introduced into the stomach, the outer end of the tube is taped to the forehead of the patient. The mouth of the tube is usually closed to prevent the leakage of gastric contents.

Indications

Diagnostic indications

- The Ryle's tube is passed to collect the gastric aspirate for acid studies.
- To diagnose pyloric stenosis, tracheoesophageal fistula and anorectal fistula.
- To collect the gastric lavage for acid fast bacillus.

Therapeutic indications

- Acute intestinal obstruction, acute peritonitis and postoperatively in case of bowel surgery for feeding purpose.
- In comatose patients for feeding and to avoid aspiration.
- Following maxillofacial injury or surgery.
- In patient who cannot take orally for/reasons like anorexia, the nasogastric tube may be used.
- For forced feeding.

Chapter 6

Tracheostomy Instruments

Amol Doiphode, Girish Thakur, Sara Ahmed

TRACHEOSTOMY TUBES

FULLER'S BIFLANGED TRACHEOSTOMY TUBE

It is a metallic tube consisting of two components, viz. an outer biflanged tube and an inner tube. The inner tube has an opening through its posterior wall. This opening allows the use of normal passages in the absence of any obstruction upwards. Thus, it helps in re-educating the patient to use normal passages during decannulation. The inner tube is always made longer than the outer tube so that the outer tube will not get blocked by secretions. This tube has no obturator because it can be introduced by simply pinching the biflanged outer tube.

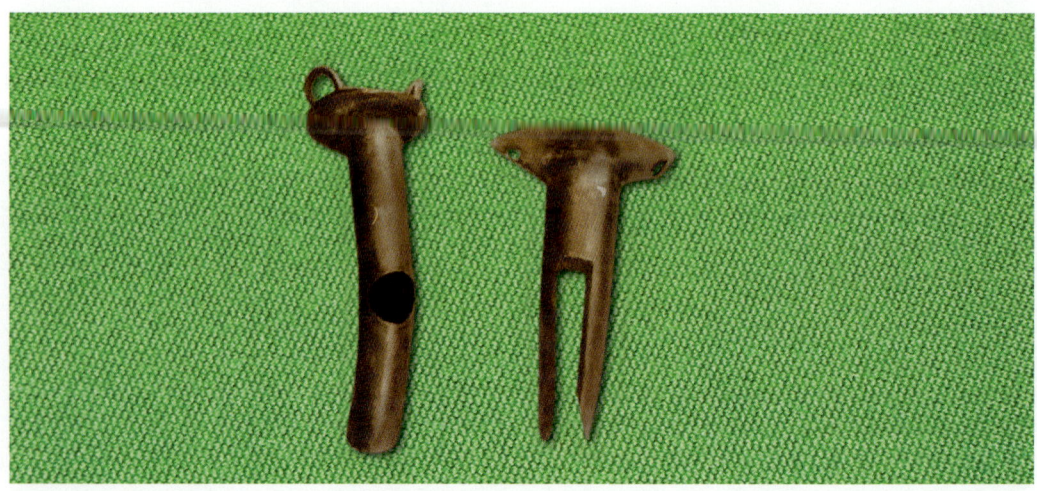

Fuller's biflanged tracheostomy tube

JACKSON'S TRACHEOSTOMY TUBE

It consists of three parts—the inner tube, the outer tube and obturator. Outer tube has a provision to lock in the inner tube. The tube is fixed in place by means of stick tapes. Outer tube is introduced along with the obturator into tracheostoma. The obturator is removed instantly and is replaced by inner tube. Inner tube is made longer than the outer so that the latter will not remain obstructed when inner tube is removed for cleaning.

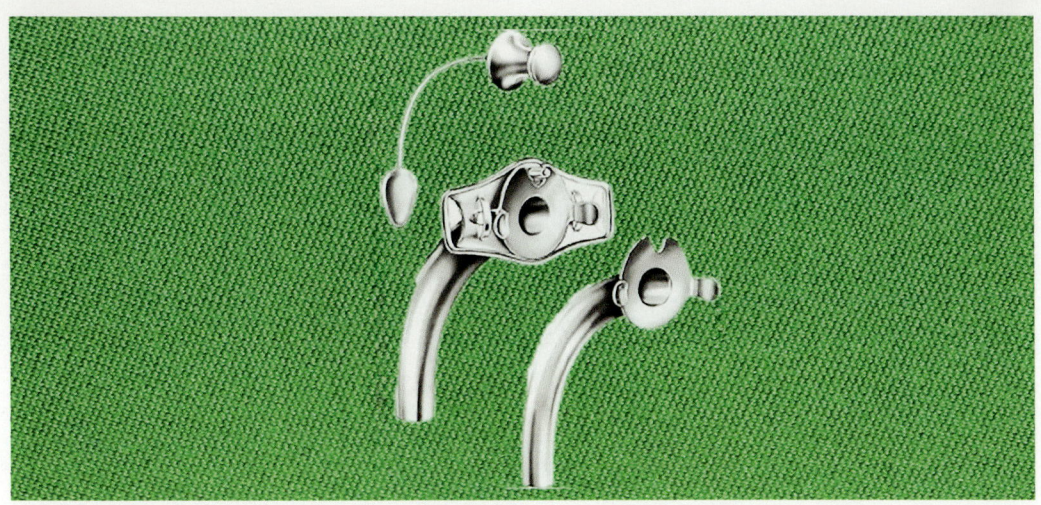

Jackson's tracheostomy tube

POLYVINYL CHLORIDE TRACHEOSTOMY TUBE

Modern tracheostomy tubes are made of plastic and are manufactured with or without an inflatable cuff. Plastic tracheostomy tubes are softer, less irritating, presterilised and disposable. A cuffed tracheostomy tube is preferred in patients who have assisted mechanical ventilation. It is essential to inflate and deflate the cuff at regular intervals to prevent pressure necrosis.

Indication

- It helps in maintenance of normal respiration in patient with obstruction in upper respiratory tract while breathing.

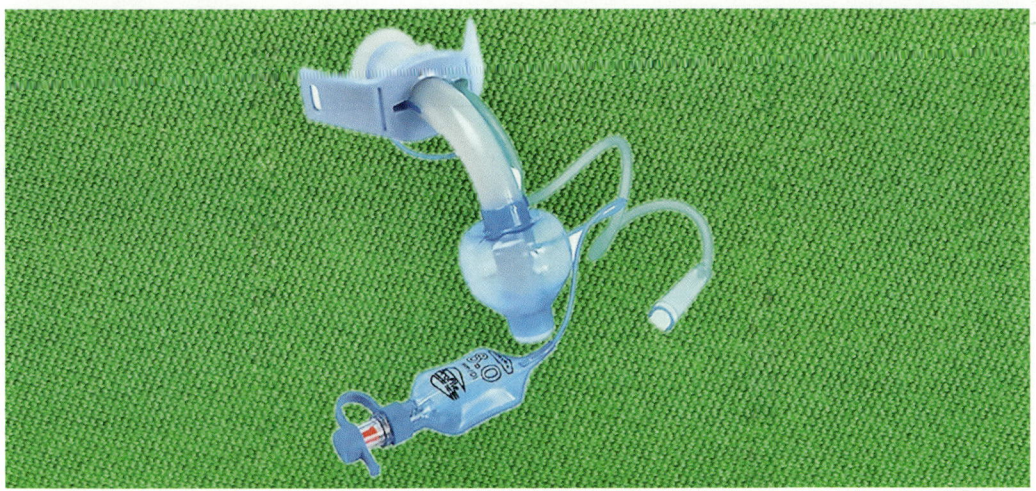

Polyvinyl chloride (PVC) tracheostomy tube

RED RUBBER ENDOTRACHEAL TUBE

Conventionally used endotracheal tube in case of emergency airway management. Available in many sizes. Made up of red soft rubber, with cuff, contains natural rubber latex along with a pilot balloon. They are nonsterile with a universal injection port.

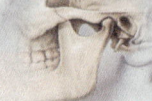

Indication

- Emergency airway management.

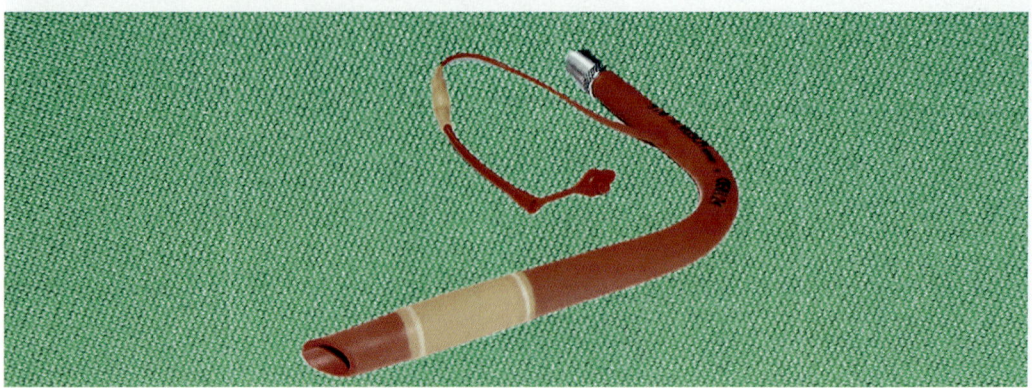

Red rubber endotracheal tube

TRACHEAL HOOK

It is slender instrument with its working end curved and sharp into a single hook.

Indications

- A tracheal hook with blunt end is used to retract thyroid isthmus upwards or downwards to expose tracheal rings.
- A tracheal hook with sharp end is applied to lower border of cricoid cartilage to stabilize the trachea and prevent its movement during respiration while making an incision in the tracheal wall.

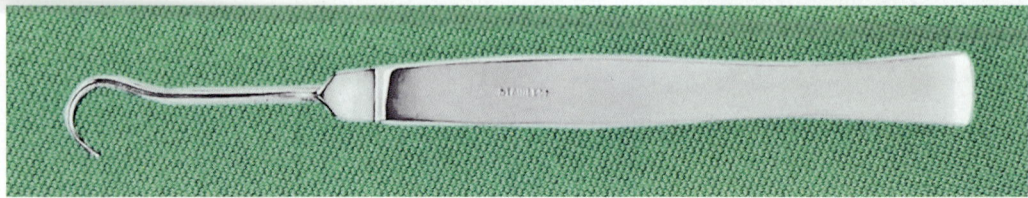

Tracheal hook

TRACHEAL DILATOR

This is an instrument with no ratchet at the non-operating end. The opening end is blunt and curved. The peculiarity of this instrument is that when its handle is opened, the operating end is closed and when the handle is closed, operating end is opened.

Indication

- Tracheal dilator is used in the post-tracheostomy period, when the tube has to be changed due to blockage. In such a situation, once the tube is removed, tracheal dilator is introduced, the opening in trachea is kept open, and the new tube is introduced.

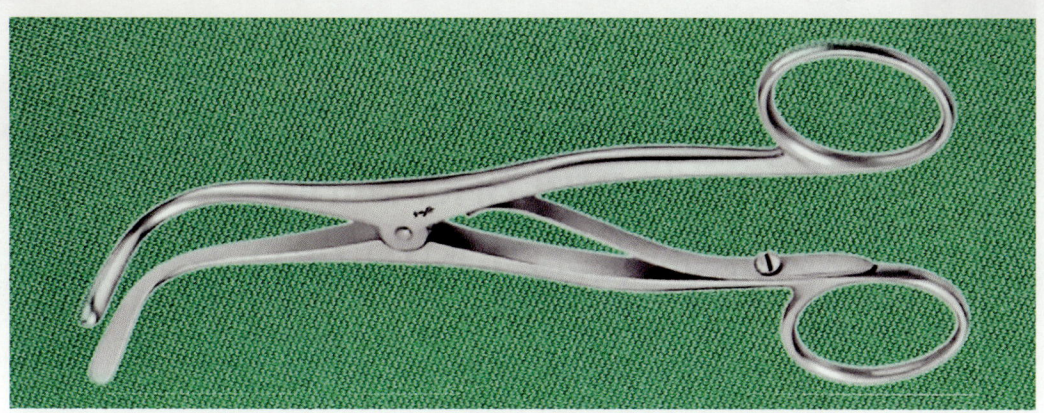

Tracheal dilator

Note: Scalpel, Artery forceps, Mosquito forceps and Langenback retractor are explained in General Surgery Instruments and Minor Oral Surgical Instruments.

Exodontia and Minor Oral Surgery Instruments

Sheeraz Badal, Sandesh Chougule

MAXILLARY ANTERIOR FORCEPS

Identifying Features

Straight, symmetrical beaks, flame shaped space present between both beaks. Beaks are broad. Broad tips close to each other.

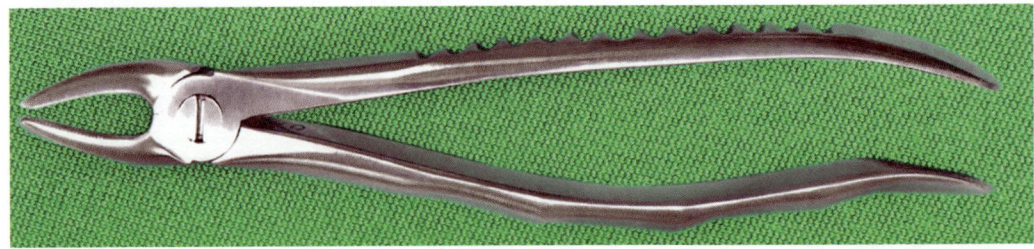

Maxillary anterior forceps

How to use?

- Beaks are inserted into buccal and palatal PDL space of the tooth with instrument parallel to long axis of the tooth.
- Movements given are primarily buccal, palatal and rotational.

Indication

Used for removal of maxillary central incisor, lateral incisor and canine teeth.

MAXILLARY PREMOLAR FORCEPS

Identifying Features

Beaks are slightly curved from base with concave side upward and towards the operator for proper access. Beaks are broad and open. Handles are slightly curved in

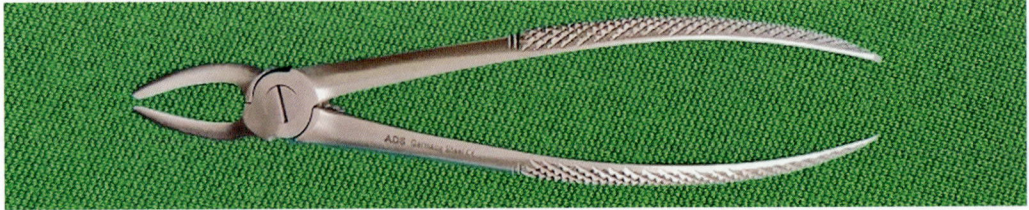

Maxillary Premolar forceps

vertical plane with convex side facing upwards. Available in paired forms as left and right.

How to use?

- Beaks are inserted into buccal and palatal PDL space of the tooth with instrument parallel to long axis of the tooth.
- Movements given are primarily buccal and palatal.

Indication

- Used for removal of maxillary premolar teeth.

MAXILLARY MOLAR FORCEPS

Identifying Features

Beaks are slightly curved upwards with concave side upwards and towards the operator. One beak is broad ended. Other beak ends in an acute point in its centre. The handle is slightly curved convex upwards and towards the operator. Inner surface of the beaks has vertical serrations for better grip. Beaks are convex on the outer surface and concave on the inner surface. These forceps are paired as for left and right.

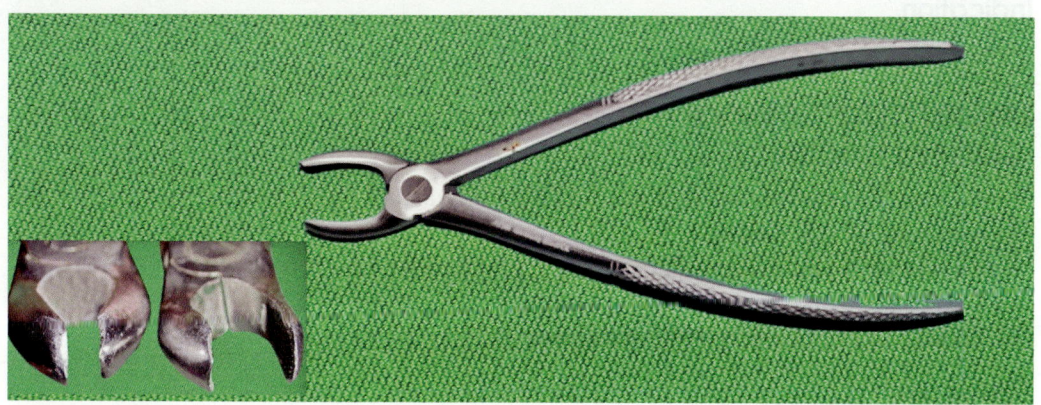

Maxillary molar forcep

How to use?

- The pointed portion of the beak goes into the furcation between the mesiobuccal and disto-buccal roots at the CEJ or cervical to it.
- The flat ended portion of the beak approximates the palatal root at or cervical to CEJ. Primarily, the movements are buccal along with palatal.

Indication

Used for removal of maxillary molar teeth.

MAXILLARY COWHORN FORCEPS

Identifying Features

Both beaks are slightly curved with concave side facing upward. Handles are slightly curved with convex side facing upward. One beak has a pointed tip. The other beak has bifid pointed tips.

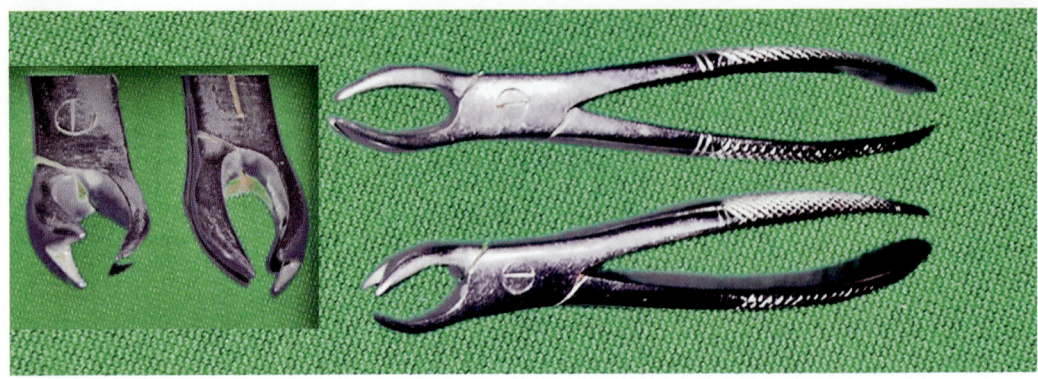

Maxillary cowhorn forceps

How to use?

- The single ended pointed beak goes into the furcation area between mesiobuccal and distobuccal roots.
- Primarily, movements are buccal along with palatal.
- The double ended beaks are used to engage the palatal root.

Indication

- Used for removal of maxillary molar teeth.

BAYONET FORCEPS OR ROOT FORCEPS

Identifying Features

- Handles are slightly curved with convex upward.
- Beaks are symmetrical.
- Each beak is acutely angulated in two planes with pointed tips.
- Tips of the beaks are closed and touching each other.
- These pairs of beaks are of two types—thin beaks and thick beaks.

How to use?

- Bayonet with thin beaks are used to remove separated individual roots.
- Bayonet with thick beaks are used to remove roots which are not separated and joined at the furcation.

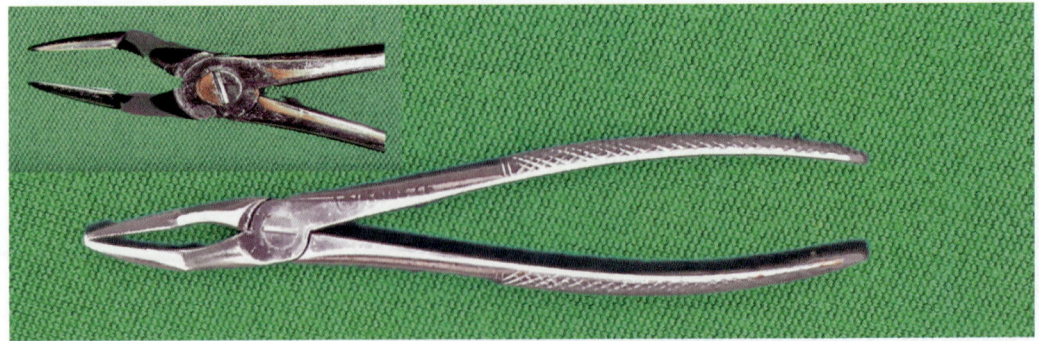

Bayonet forceps or root forceps

Indication

- It is used to remove the maxillary root stumps.

MAXILLARY THIRD MOLAR FORCEPS

Identifying Features

- Handles are slightly curved with convex side facing upward.
- Beaks are symmetrical.
- Beaks are short, wide with smooth rounded tips.

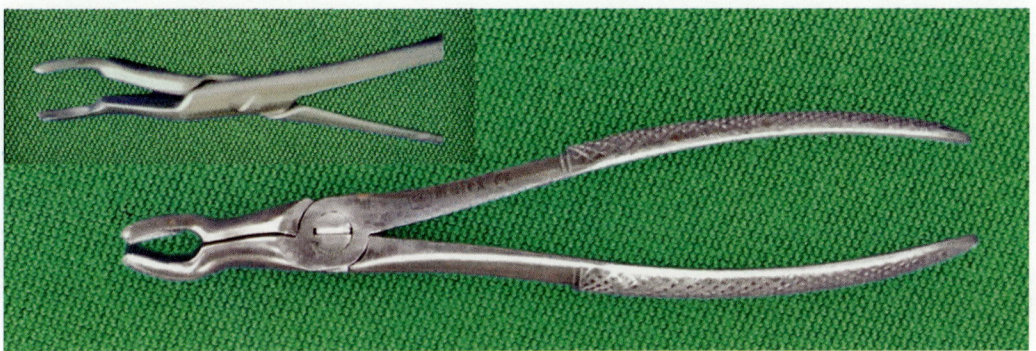

Maxillary Third Molar Forceps

How to use?

- Each beak is approximated closely at the CEJ.
- Primarily, the movements are buccal along with palatal.

Indication

- It is used to remove the maxillary 3rd molars.

MANDIBULAR ANTERIOR FORCEPS

Identifying Features

- Handles are parallel to each other in vertical plane, beaks are at an angle of about 90 degrees to handles, rivet like joint is seen, beaks are symmetrical. Beaks have broad ends with tips touching each other.

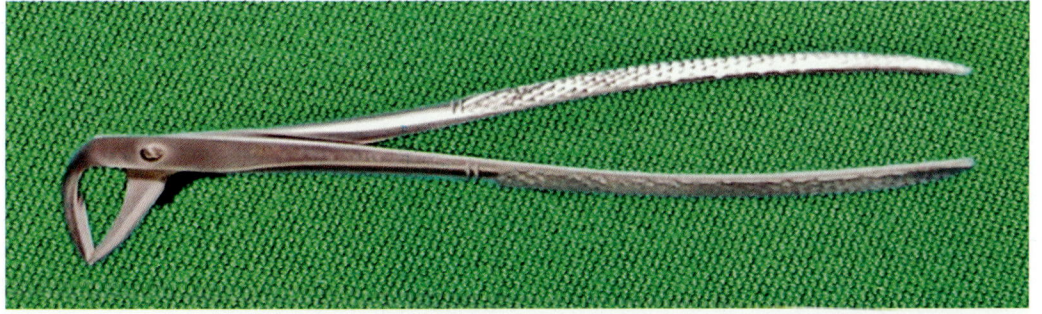

Mandibular anterior forceps

How to use?

- Beaks face downward, beak closer to the operator is inserted into the PDL in close approximation with buccal surface of the root.
- The other beak is inserted into the PDL in close approximation with lingual surface of the root.
- Primarily, movements are buccal along with lingual. It can also be used for removal of single or separated roots.

Indication

- Used for removal of mandibular central incisors, lateral incisors and canines.

MANDIBULAR PREMOLAR FORCEP

Identifying Features

- Handles are parallel to each other in vertical plane.
- Beaks are at an angle of about 90° to handle.
- Rivet like joint is seen, beaks are symmetrical.
- Beaks have broad ends with tips not touching each other.

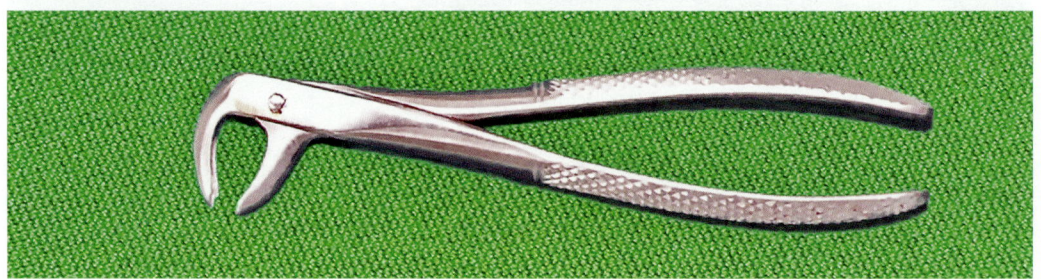

Mandibular premolar forcep

How to use?

- Beaks face downwards, beak closer to the operator is inserted into the PDL in close approximation with buccal surface of the root.
- The other beak is inserted into the PDL in close approximation with lingual surface of the root, primarily, movements are buccal along with lingual.

Indication

- Used for removal of mandibular premolars.

MEAD FORCEPS/MANDIBULAR MOLAR FORCEPS

Identifying Features

- Handles are parallel to each other in vertical plane.
- Each beak has a centre pointed tip and do not touch each other.
- Serrations are present vertically on the inner surfaces of the beaks.

How to use?

- Beaks face downwards and the one closer to the operator is inserted into the PDL in close approximation with buccal surface of the root at CEJ.

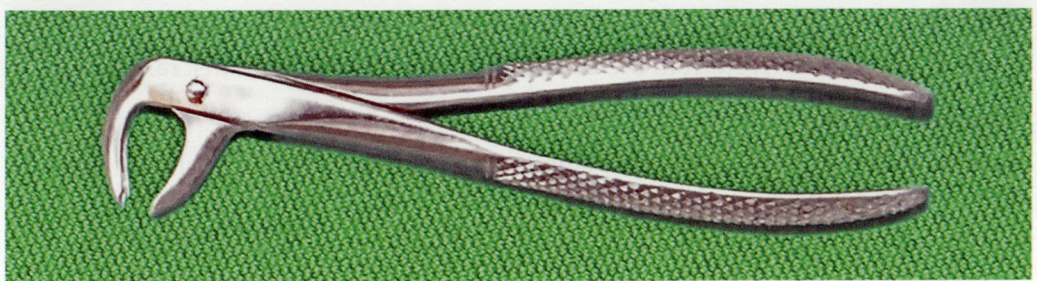

Mead forceps/mandibular molar forceps

- The other beak is inserted into the PDL in close approximation with lingual surface of the root at CEJ and near the furcation.
- The movements given are buccal along with lingual.

Indication

- Used for removal of mandibular molars.

COWHORN FORCEPS

Identifying Features

- Handles are parallel to each other in vertical plane.
- Each beak is thinner than mead forceps with a pointed tip.
- Beaks do not touch each other, oval space is vertically present between the beaks separating them.

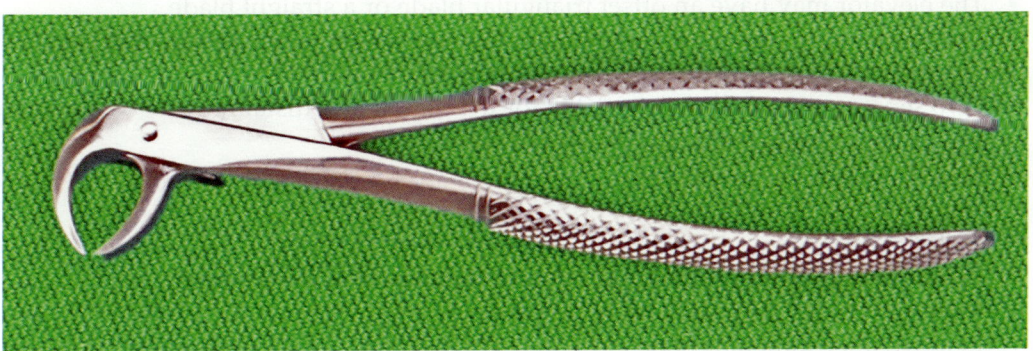

Cowhorn forceps

How to use?

- Beaks face downwards, beak closer to the operator is inserted into the PDL in close approximation with buccal surface into the furcation.
- The other beak is inserted into the PDL in close approximation with lingual surface into the furcation, movements given are buccal along with lingual.

Indication

Used for removal of mandibular molars which are grossly carious with intact furcation.

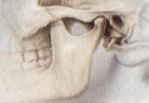

ELEVATORS

Word 'elevator' is derived from the Latin word 'elevare' which means 'raise'.

Dental Elevators

A dental instrument used for removing teeth or the roots of teeth which cannot be gripped with a forceps.

Parts

Blade, shank and handle.

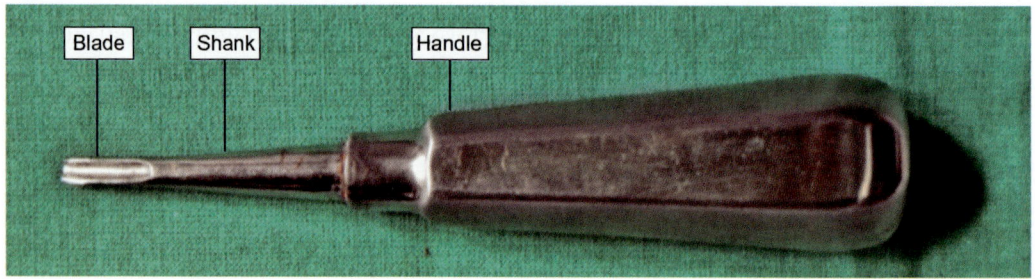

Blade and shank differ with different dental elevators.
Handle has two designs
- Heavy pear shaped
- Crossbar: Right angles to the shank

Identifying Features

- The elevator may have an offset triangular blade or a straight blade.
- The working tip may be angulated and has one concave and another flat surface. The concave surface is the working side and it faces the tooth/root to be removed.
- Two separate elevators are available for the mesial and distal roots.
  For example, winter cryer, crossbar elevator.
- Handle is heavy pear shaped.

Indications

- Luxate teeth from the surrounding bone making extractions easier.
- Remove broken/surgically sectioned roots.
- Remove inter-radicular bone.

Rules for use of Elevators

- Use only where indicated.
  For example, apexo elevator is used for elevation of conical root pieces.
- Use finger guard to avoid injury to the adjacent soft tissue.
- Use judiciously near maxillary sinus region, inferior alveolar nerve and other vital structures.

NEVER

- **Never** use adjacent tooth as fulcrum, unless to be extracted during the same sitting.

PRINCIPLES OF DENTAL ELEVATION

There are three principles of dental elevation:
- Lever principle
- Wedge principle
- Wheel and axle principle

A. Lever Principle

The position of fulcrum is between the effort (E) and the resistance arm (R).

   The effort arm on one side of the fulcrum must be longer than the resistance arm.

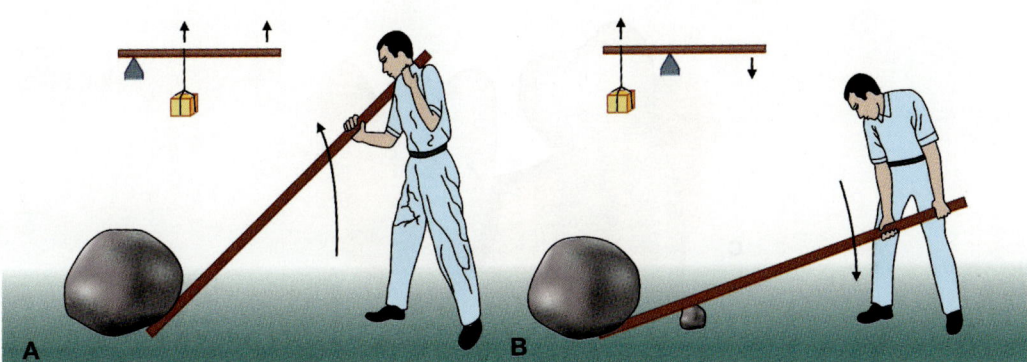

Types of Lever

- *First class lever:* Fulcrum is located in between the input effort and the output load.
- *Second class lever:* Fulcrum is located at the other end of the bar, opposite to input, with the output load at a point between these two forces.
- *Third class lever:* The input effort is higher than the output load, which is different from the first-class and second-class levers.

Mechanical advantage:

R: Resistance arm and E: Effort arm.

$$\text{Resistance Arm} \times \text{Short Arm} = \text{Effort Arm} \times \text{Long Arm}$$

Long Arm = 3/4th of the total arm

Short Arm = 1/4th of the total arm

$$R \times 1/4th = E \times 3/4th$$

   R = 3E

R/E = 3/1

Mechanical advantage = **3**

For example, straight elevator.

Used for luxation of teeth which are impacted, malposed or badly carious.
   The blade has a concave surface on one side that faces the tooth to be elevated.

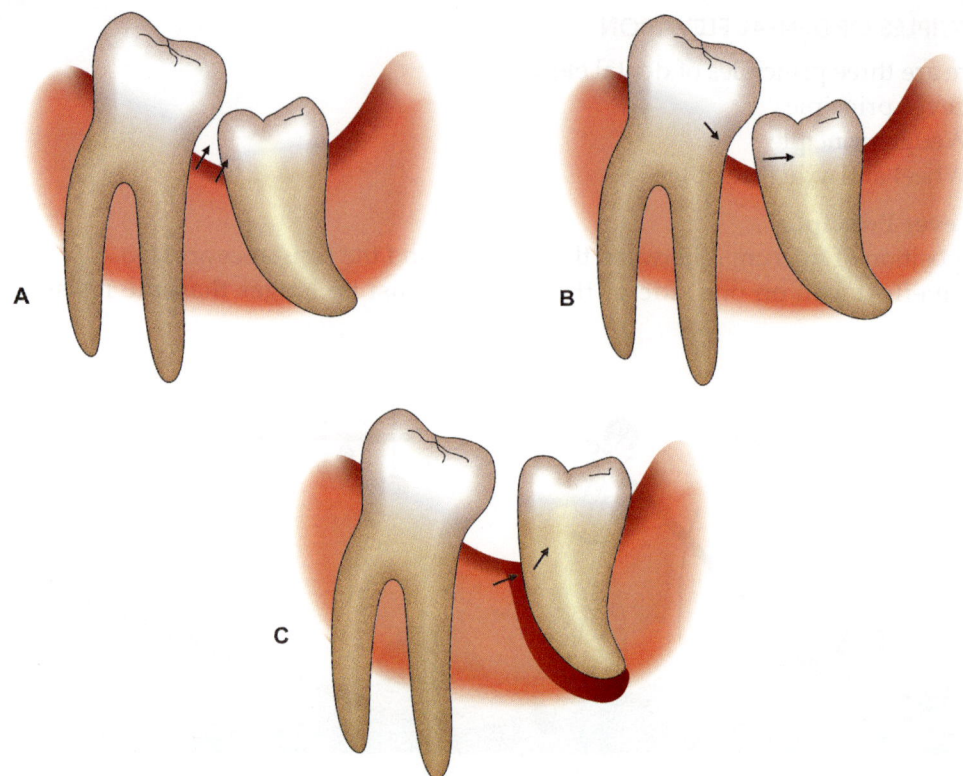

B. Wedge Principle

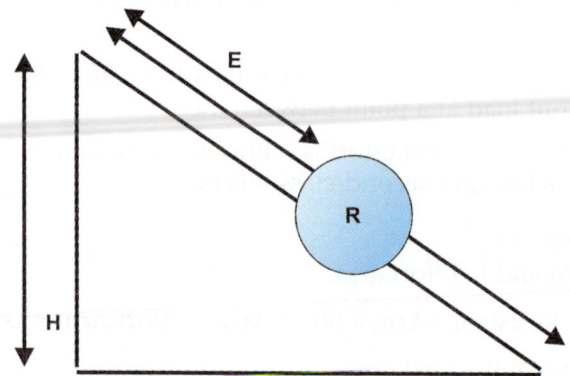

R: Resistance, E: Effort, L: Length and H: Height

Formula for wedge: Effort × Length = Resistance × Height

$$E \times L = R \times H$$

where, L = 10 mm, H = 4 mm

Mechanical advantage = R/E = 10/4 = **2.5**

For example, apexo elevator.

- Apexo elevators are the specially designed elevators based only on wedge principle.
- The wedge elevator is forced between the root of the tooth and the investing bony tissue parallel to the long axis of the root.

- Mostly used in conjunction with lever and/or wheel and axle principle.
- The wedge is a movable inclined plane, which overcomes large resistance at right angles to applied force.
- The sharper the angle of the wedge, the lesser the effort required.

C. Wheel and axle principle: (Modified form of lever principle)

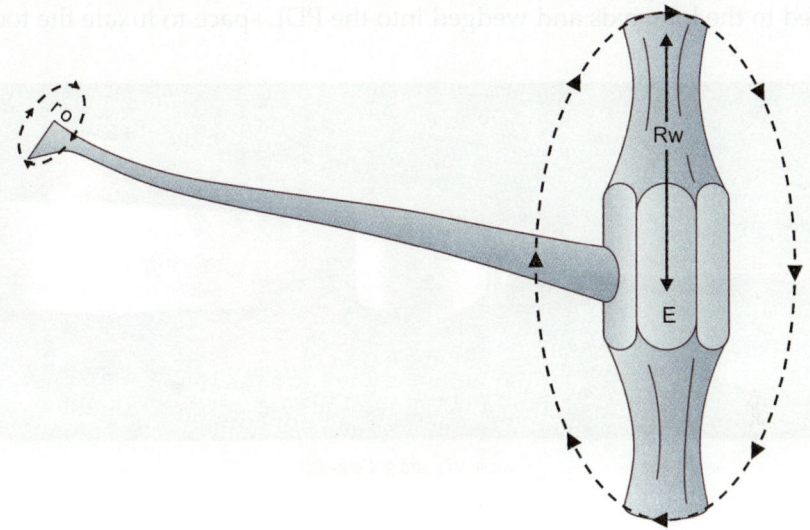

Effort × radius of wheel = Resistance × radius of axel

$$E \times Rw = R \times ra$$

where, $Rw = 42$; $ra = 9$

Mechanical advantage = $Rw/ra = 42/9 = $ **4.6**

For example, crossbar elevator

- The effort is applied to the circumference of a wheel which turns the axel to raise a weight.
- The force applied at tip of elevator to elevate the tooth/ root is 4.6 times more than the force applied at the handle.

STRAIGHT ELEVATOR

Most commonly used for luxation of teeth. Blade is having concave surface on one side, facing to the tooth to be elevated. Angled straight elevator is used for good access to posterior aspects of the oral cavity.

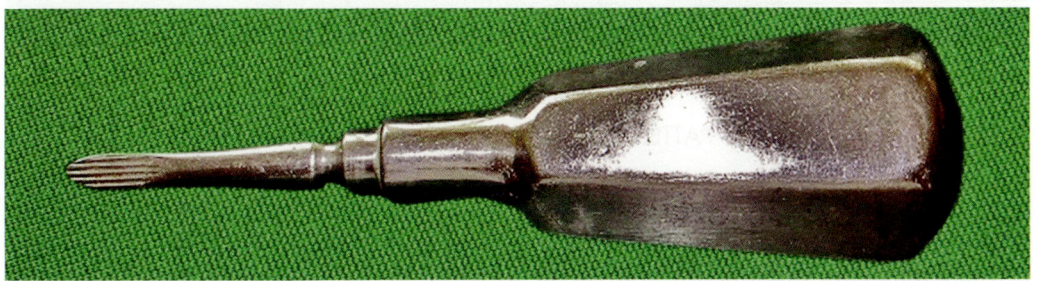

Straight elevator

COUPLAND'S STRAIGHT ELEVATOR

It has large pear-shaped handle and a straight shank. Blade has a concave/convex surface and an inclined plane. It has sharp and straight tip. Used in impacted/malaligned teeth. Works on wedge and 1st order lever principle.

- Applied at 45p to long axis of the tooth with concavity facing the tooth.
- Crest of the interseptal bone is used as fulcrum.
- Applied to the long axis and wedged into the PDL space to luxate the tooth.

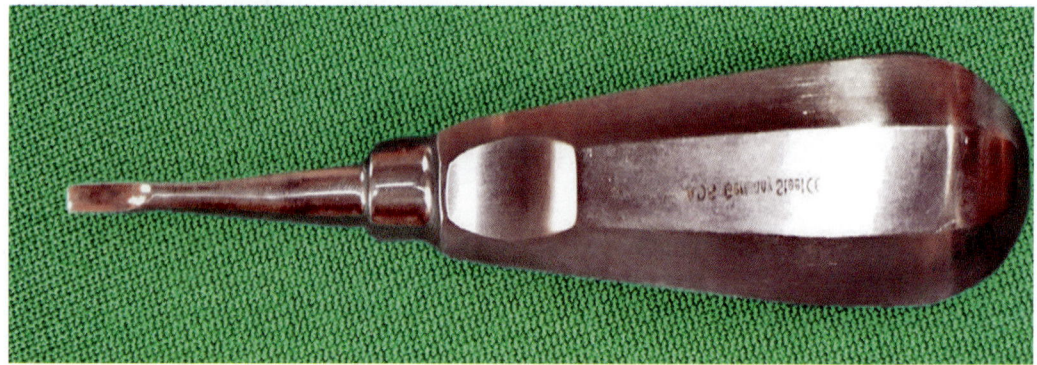

Coupland's straight elevator

APEXO ELEVATOR

It has an 'offset'/angulated blade with a large pear-shaped handle. Blade ends have sharp pointed tips. It is available in pairs, i.e. mesial and distal. Remove root fragments fractured at the apical third of the root. It works on Wedge principle.

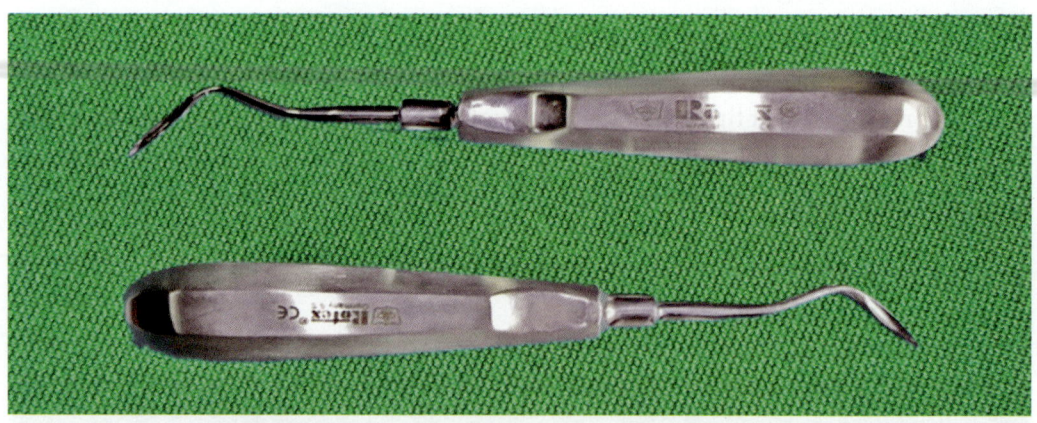

Apexo elevator

WINTER CRYER (STRAIGHT PATTERN)

It has an 'offset' blade at an angle to the shank and the blades are curved and triangular. Its handle is heavy and pear shaped. It is available in pairs. It is used in impacted molar surgery, removal of fractured root tips of maxillary molars and erupted maxillary molars. Bur hole can be drilled onto the tooth to engage the tip and acquire the purchase point.

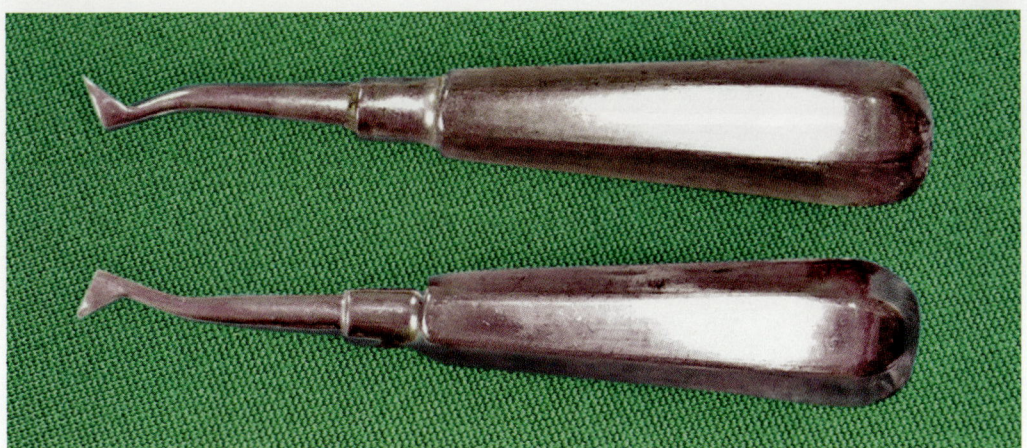

Winter cryer (straight pattern)

WINTER CRYER (CROSSBAR PATTERN)

It has an 'offset blade' design where the blade is at an angle to the shank and handle. Working tip is triangular and at an angle to the shank. The blade has a convex and a flat surface which is the working surface and is placed facing the tooth to be elevated and works on wheel and axle and with wedge principles.

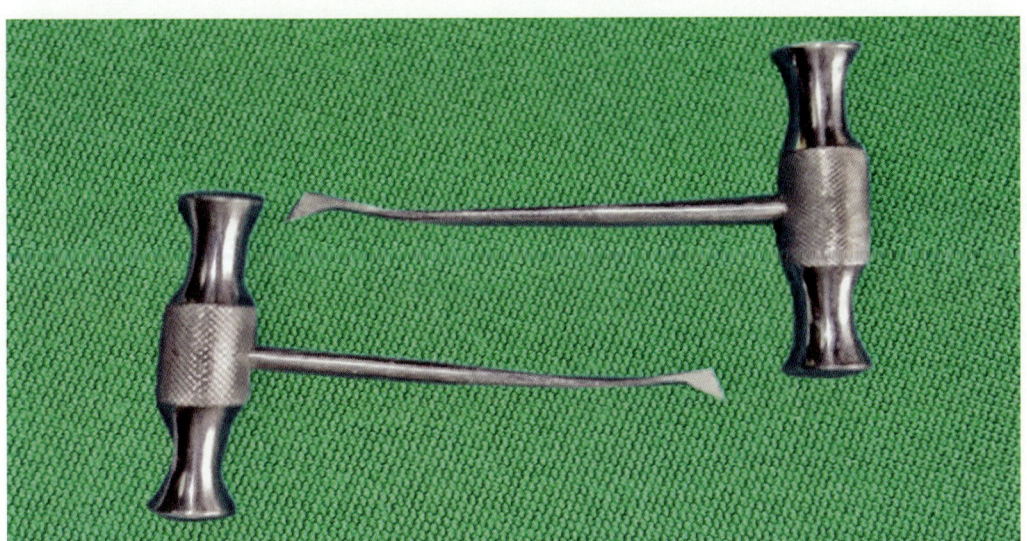

Winter cryer (crossbar pattern)

DIAGNOSTIC INSTRUMENTS

MOUTH MIRROR

Synonym—Odontoscope

PARTS OF MOUTH MIRROR
- Working end, shank, handle

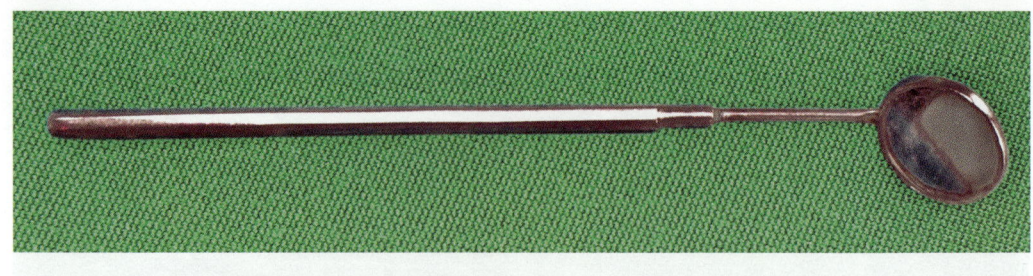

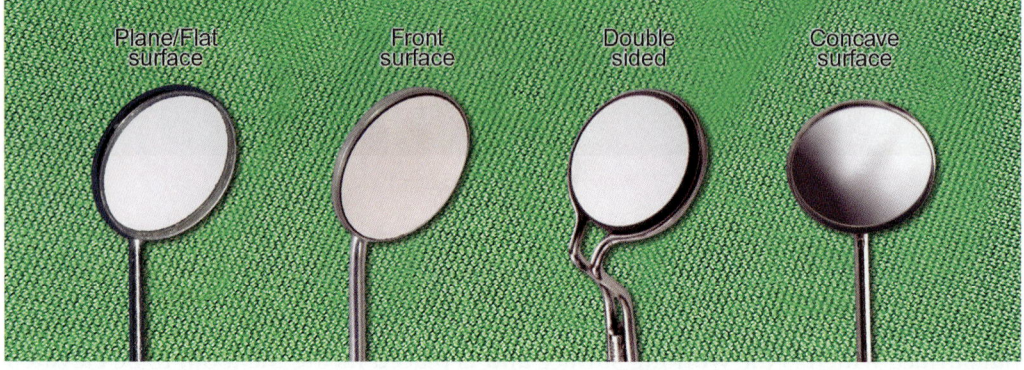

Minor oral surgical instruments mouth mirror

Types of Mouth Mirror

a. **Based on material:** Stainless steel and plastic (plastic mirrors are disposable)

b. **Based on size:** No. 1, No. 2, No. 3, No. 4, No. 5, No. 6

(Most commonly used are no. 4 and no. 5)

c. **Based on reflecting surface of the mirror**

Flat (Plane, Regular) Surface Mirrors
- They have reflective surfaces (silver coating) on the back of the glass. This gives the image—"a ghost image". It reflects only once to give a clear view free of distortion and may produce double image.
- This type of mouth mirror is used in the disposable models.

Concave Surface Mirrors
- This type of mirror is used to magnify the image, and it makes the visible area look larger to provide a better image of the area for diagnosis, especially the gums, and areas between the teeth and gums.

Front Surface Mirrors
- They produce a perfect, accurate, and an image free of any distortion or change in size.
- They have reflective coatings (rhodium) on top of the glass, this coating eliminates the "ghost image".

DIAGNOSTIC PROBE
Probe is derived from a Latin word "Probo" which means "to test".

Parts of Probe

a. Working end
b. Shank
c. Handle

Types

a. Straight probe
b. Williams' graduated probe

Indications

A. Straight Probe

- To detect carious lesions.
- To check tooth mobility.
- To check margins of existing fillings.

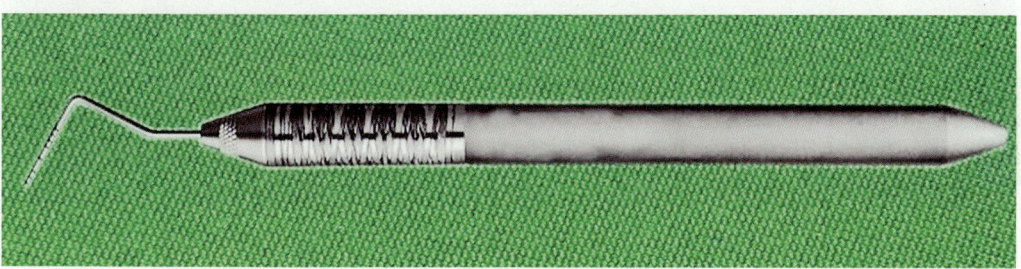
Straight probe

B. Williams graduated probe

- To detect bleeding on probing.
- To detect and measure periodontal pocket depth
- To measure dimensions of small lesions.

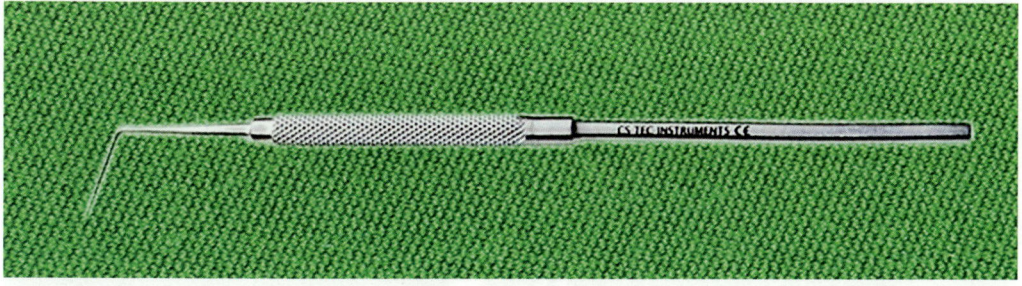
Williams graduated probe

EXPLORER

Parts

a. Working end
b. Shank
c. Handle

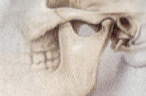

Types

Some explorers are specially designed such as,

a. Single ended
b. Double ended
  i. Orbans
  ii. Pigtail
  iii. Shepherd's hook

Many instruments have explorer at one end and probe on the other end.

Indications

- Explorers are generally used to examine incipient caries, subgingival calculus, and furcation.
- Explorers like pigtail are used to examine interproximal areas of teeth.

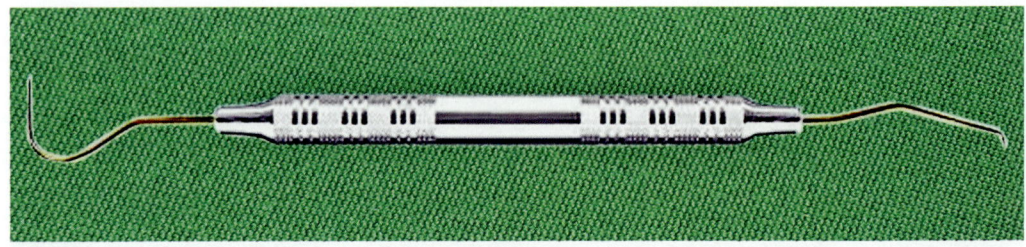

Explorer

TWEEZER

Synonyms: Cotton forceps, college plier

Parts

a. Two long arms
b. Locking device

Locking device is used to maintain beaks in closed position until released.

Advantage: Avoid unnecessary anxiety of the operator at the possibility of slippage.

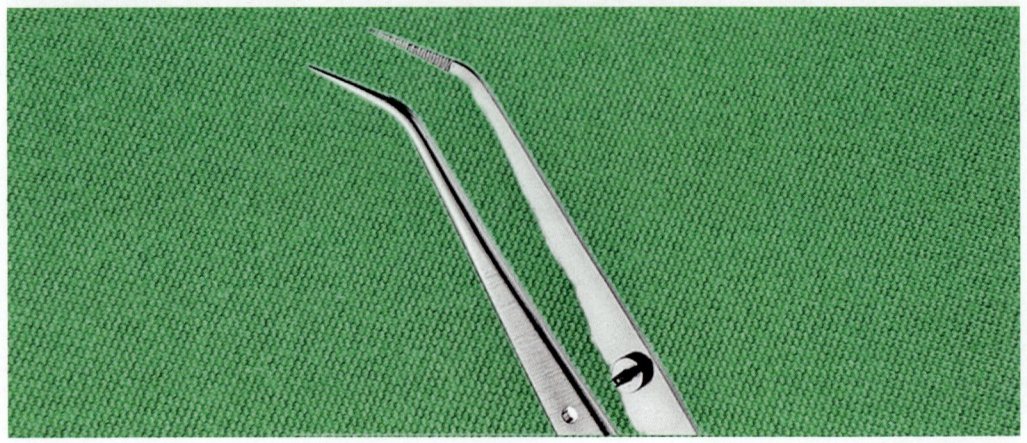

Tweezer

Indications

- To carry cotton rolls and sponge pellets to and/ or around the oral cavity.
- To carry saliva soaked cotton from the oral cavity to waste disposable units.

CUTTING INSTRUMENTS

SCALPEL/SURGEON'S KNIFE

How to use?

- **Pen grip:** It is used for delicate work, hold the handle between the thumb, middle and ring finger.
- Put the index finger on the back of the blade for better control of pressure and movements.
- **Table knife grip:** It is used to divide skin and cut through layers below it for abscess. Always hold in pen grasp.
- Blade should be held with the help of needle holder or an artery forceps while fitting the blade to the handle.

Scalpel Blade Remover

It is a specially designed instrument to safely remove blade from handle and avoid inadvertent injury to operator.

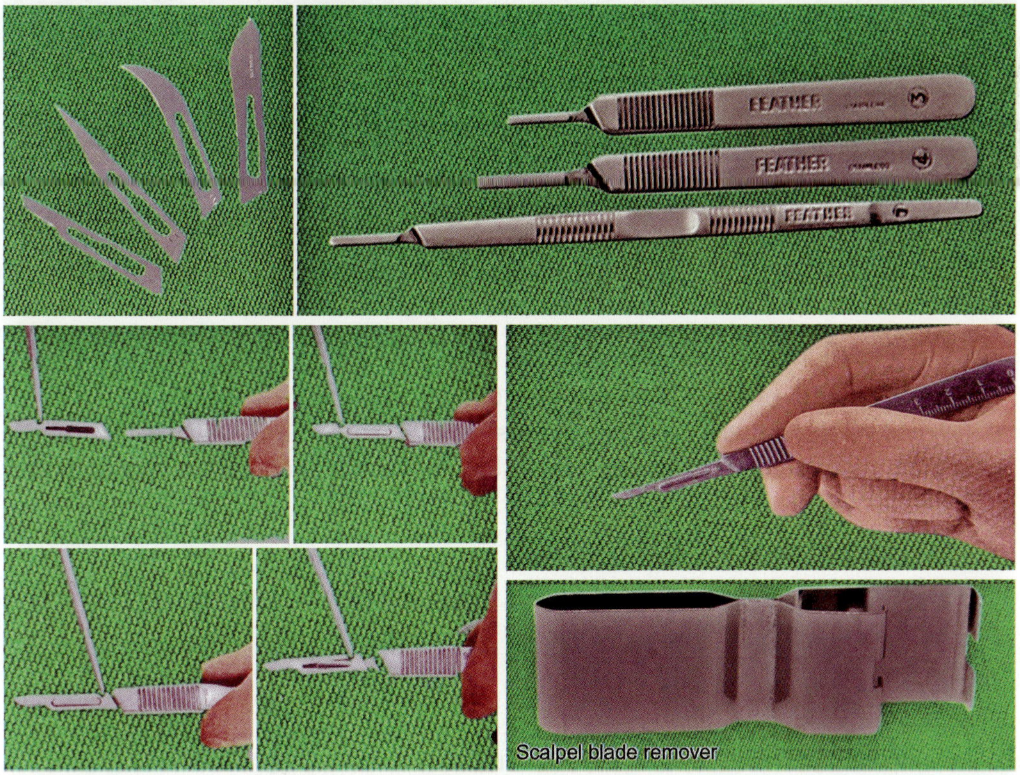

Scalpel blade remover

Scalpel/surgeon's knife

Parts of scalpel:

a. Blade.

b. Handle.

Types of Bard Parker Handle

- BP handle no. 3, 4, 7, BP handle no. 3 is used with blade no. 11, 12 and 15.
- BP handle no. 4 is used with blade no. 10.
- BP handle no. 7 is used with blade no. 15.

Types of Surgical Blades

Surgical blades no. 10, 11, 12, 15.

Indications for Different Surgical Blades

- Blade no. 10: Used for large skin, muscle and mucosal incisions.
- Blade no. 11: Used for stab incision for draining an abscess, precision cutting, stripping the tissue
- Blade no. 12: It is hook shaped. Used for mucogingival procedures and also in posterior aspects of teeth/maxillary tuberosity.
- Blade no. 15: Most commonly used for intraoral incisions.

CHISEL

Parts: Working blade, shank and handle.

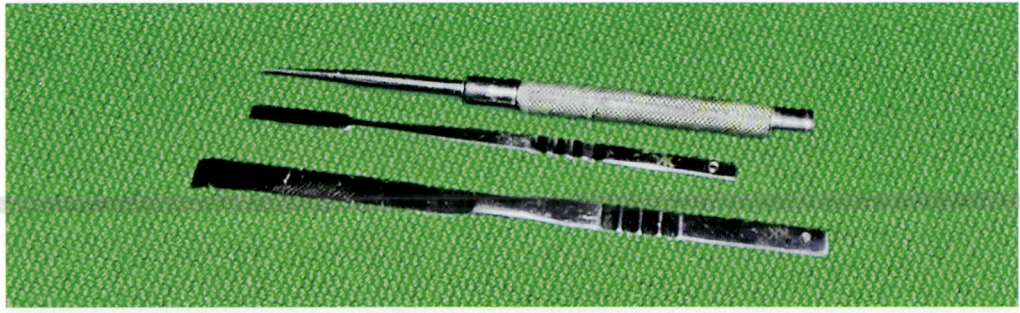

Chisel

Types of Chisel

- Based on width of blade: 5 mm, 6 mm, 10 mm, 15 mm
- Edge of working tip has a bevel on one side unlike osteotome which is bibevelled.
- It is preferably about 1/4th inch in width and handle may be 7 inches long and teflon coated.

How to use?

- For smoothing of bone the bevel is kept facing the bone, whereas to cut the bone it is kept facing away from the bone.

Indications

- To cut the bone
- To chip off bone in transalveolar extraction
- For odontectomy.

SURGICAL MALLET (MEAD'S)

Parts: Handle and working end.

Types: Teflon coated and non-teflon coated.

- It is similar to a hammer, teflon coated mallet imparts less shock to the patient and it is less noisy.

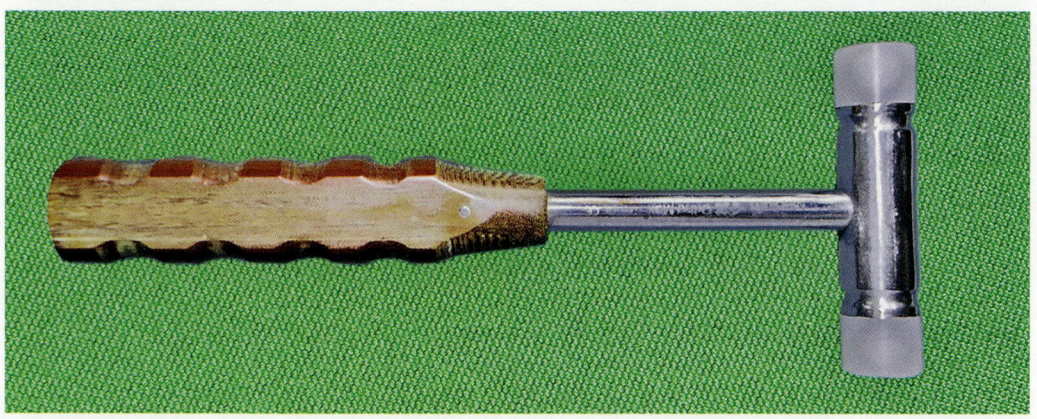

Surgical mallet (mead's)

How to use?

- To be effective mallet, it should be used in loose free swinging movement of the wrist with maximum pressure of 5 to 7 pounds.
- Usually, a 6 inches and 255 gm in weight mallet is used in oral surgical procedures.

Indication

- Used for giving controlled taps on chisel/osteotome/bone gouge.

SURGICAL BURS

Parts of burs:

a. Head
b. Shank
c. Handle

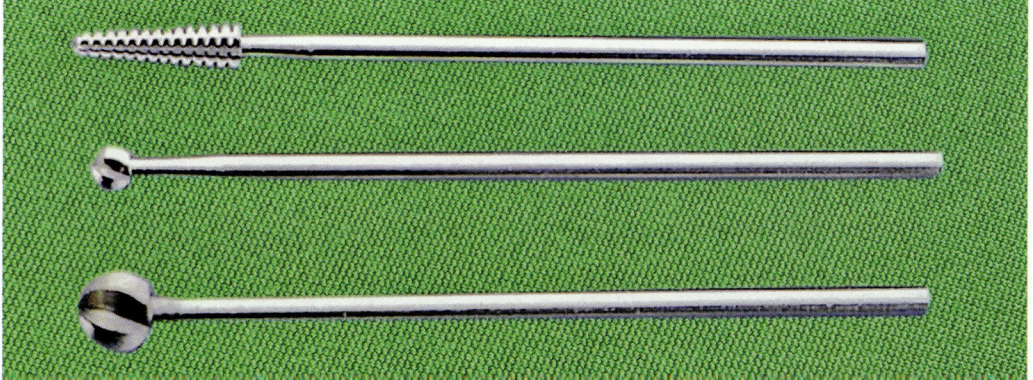

Surgical burs

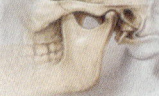

They are made of stainless steel/carbide and available in different shapes and lengths.

Types of Burs

- **Based on shapes of the burs:**

  A. Round bur   B. Straight bur

  C. Fissure bur

- The head of bur should be at least 7 mm in length so that an adequate depth of cut can be made before the wider shank (2.5 mm) engages the tooth.

Indications

- To aid in bone removal or splitting the tooth during surgical removal of tooth.
- To round off sharp margins after extractions/minor surgical procedures and during alveoloplasty.
- To make bony windows for access to cystic cavities and release bony ankylotic mass.
- To perform osteotomy cuts and resection of jaws.

Precautions

- Irrigation of the bur with sterile saline during bone cutting is essential.
- To avoid bone damage due to overheating.
- To lubricate and clean bur blades.

SURGICAL HANDPIECE

Straight micromotor handpiece is used either by attaching it to the dental chair tubing or can be used separately by using 'control-box'. The maximum speed that can be achieved with straight handpiece is 30,000 rpm. It is used along with long shank drill bit or bur.

Indications

- Fracture fixation procedures in which a drill bit is attached to the straight handpiece to drill holes before plate fixation.
- For making osteotomy cuts during orthognathic surgery.
- It is also used with round bur for smoothening the bony margins.

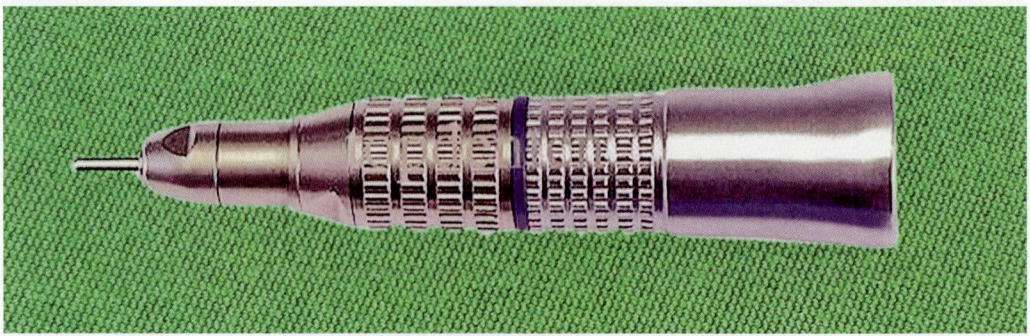

Surgical handpiece

ELEVATORS AND RETRACTORS

RIGHT ANGLED MOON'S RETRACTOR

Parts: Working end and handle.

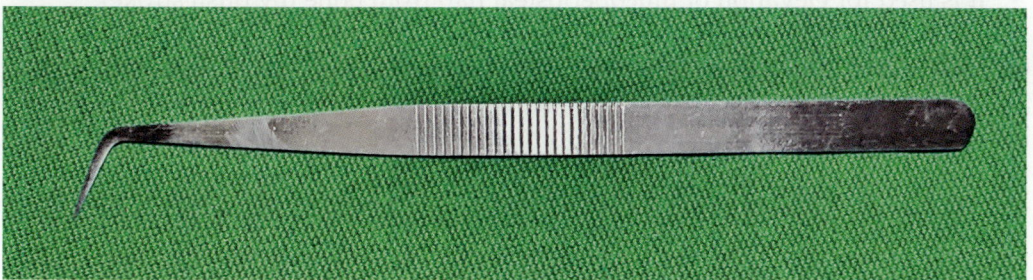

Right angled moon's retractor

Types

- Gingival tissue retractor.
- Flat handle and blade perpendicular to the handle.
- It has narrow working edge which is blunt and with rounded tip.
- Retraction is needed for good accessibility and vision.

Indications

- To check for the effectiveness of local anesthetic prior to any procedure.
- To transect gingival fibers attached to the tooth
- To check bony socket after extraction for remnants of root piece.

MOLT'S NO. 9 PERIOSTEAL ELEVATOR

Molt's periosteal elevator has one pointed end and the other end is broad and blunt with convex surafce outside and concavity on inner side of blade.

Parts: Two woking ends and a handle connecting them.

Indications

- Pointed end used to release the dental papilla around teeth (by prying motion).
- Broad end used for elevating the mucoperiosteal flap form bone (by push stroke).

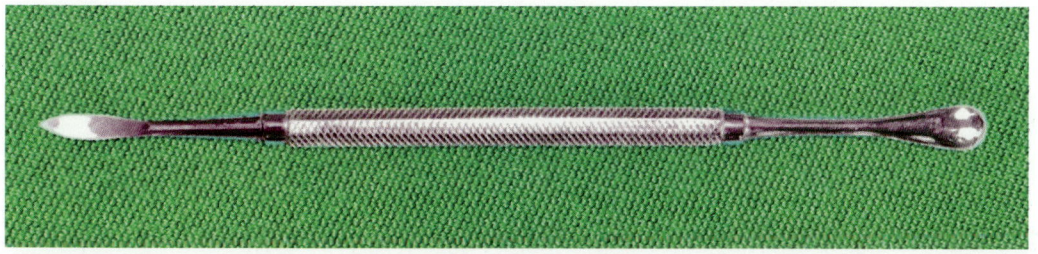

Molt's no. 9 periosteal elevator

HOWARTH'S PERIOSTEAL ELEVATOR

It has one broad end similar to that of the molt's periosteal elevator but the other end is rectangular with right angled sharp extension which is called rugine end.

Indication

- It is used for elevation of mucoperiosteal flap from bone (by push stroke).

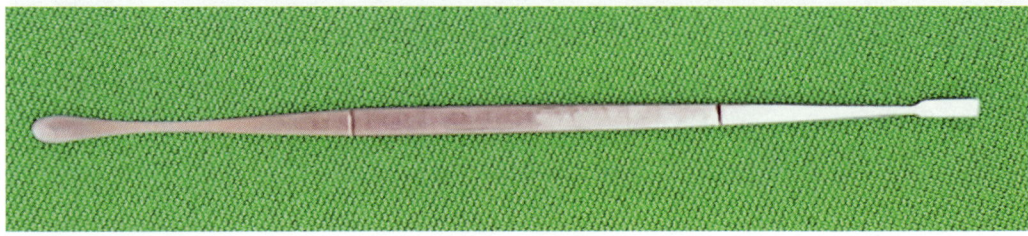

Howarth's periosteal elevator

AUSTIN'S RETRACTOR

- It is short angulated instrument with working end has forked, half moon, and regular pattern.

Indication

- This is the most commonly used instrument for the retraction of flap during removal of impacted third molar and periodontal surgery.

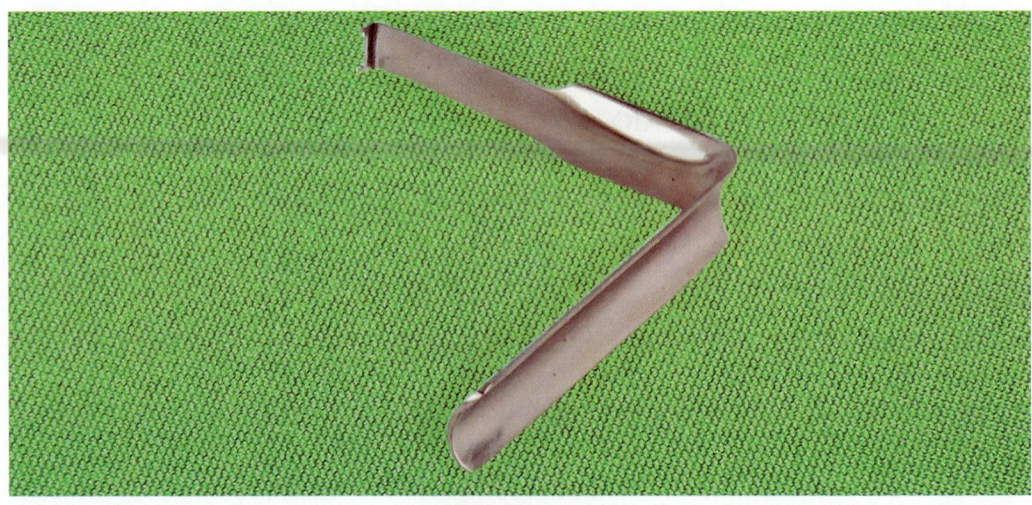

Austin's retractor

MINNESOTA RETRACTOR

It is broad retractor with flat working end curved at two planes.

Indication

- It is commonly used instrument for the retraction of flap during removal of impacted third molar and periodontal surgery.

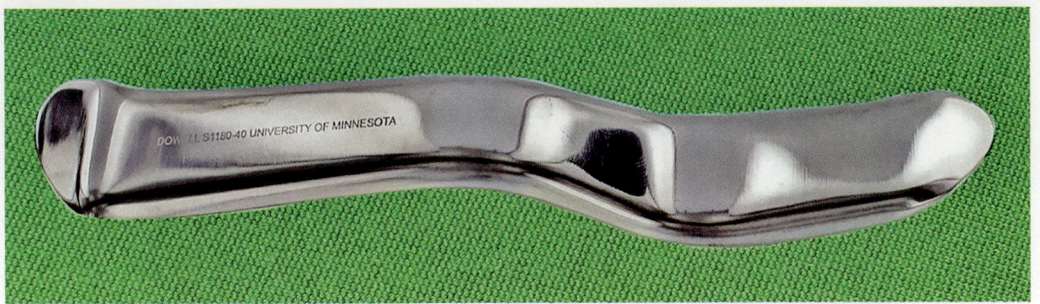

Minnesota retractor

CHEEK RETRACTOR

Types

- Metal and plastic
- Single ended and double ended
- It is flexible with curve at working end to accommodate the corner of lip.

Indication

- It is used for retraction of lips and cheeks during operative procedure.

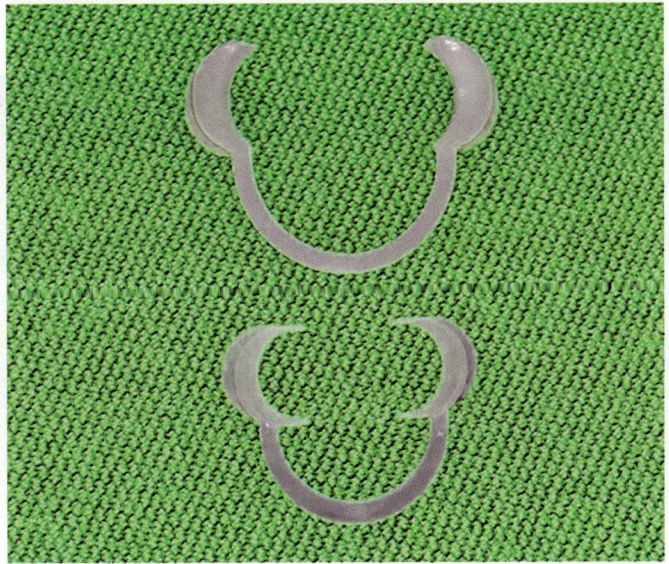

Cheek retractor

IRRIGATION AND DEBRIDEMENT

STEEL BOWL

Stainless steel bowls are available in various sizes and are autoclavable.

Indication

- Stainless steel bowl is used to carry irrigation solutions like saline and betadine in preoperative, intraoperative and postoperative procedures.

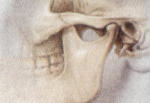

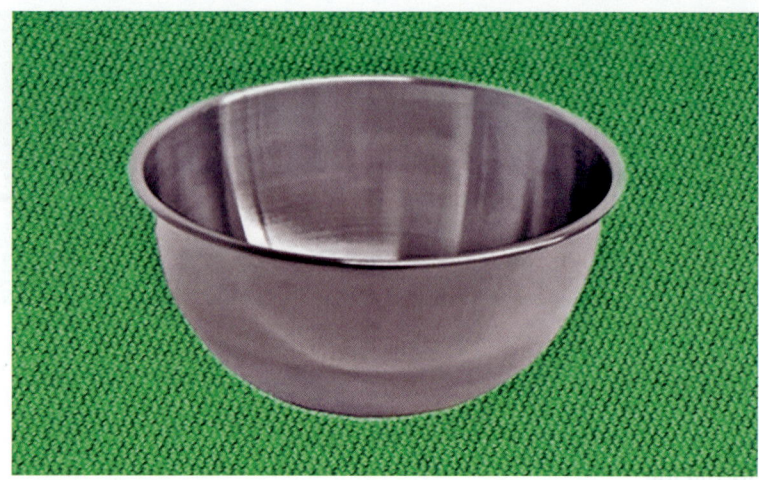

Steel bowl

BONE CURETTES

Always held in "thumb and palm" grasp and used in "pull (scrape)" stroke. It has two angulated scooped working ends and a handle connecting them that bears serrations for grip. It is used unidirectionally with a "pull stroke" (push stroke causes burnishing and crushing of bone).

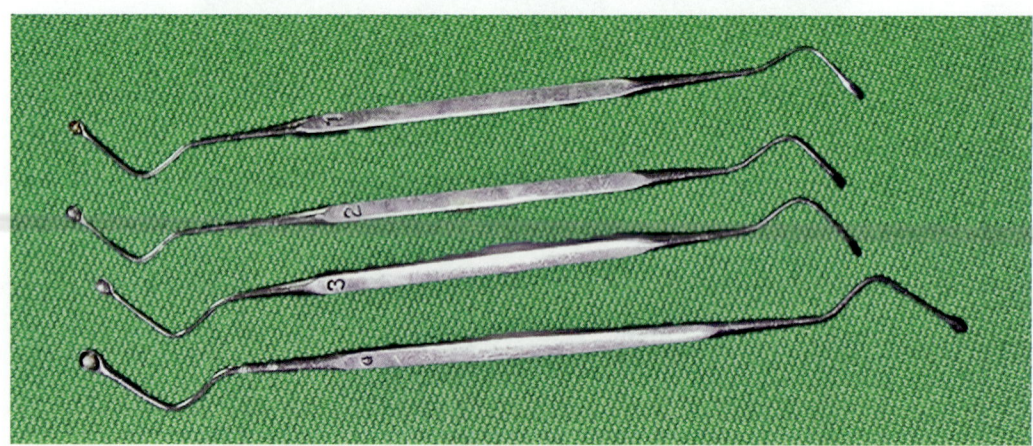

Bone curettes

Indications

- It is used to curette the granulation tissue and also cystic lining.
- It is used for final smoothening of bony socket before suturing.

VOLKMANN'S SCOOP

Types:
  i. Single ended
 ii. Double ended

Working edges are more deepened/pronounced as a scoop.

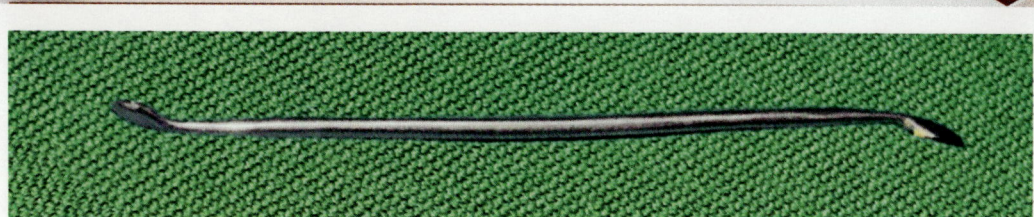

Volkmann's scoop

Indications

- To scrape the contents of a cavity similar to curette and to collect the contents from a sinus tract, chronic abscess cavity or fistula.
- To curette bony cavities formed by cystic/tumorous lesions or osteomyelitic lesions.
- To scoop out the cancellous bone for grafting and to introduce graft material / antiseptic powder into the surgical area.

SUCTION CANNULA

Types

i. Disposable and non-disposable.
ii. Metal and plastic.

Surgical suction has smaller orifice than the type used in dentistry. It has a blade on the handle for better control and a hole to control the suction speed. A stylet is provided to clean the lumen, if there is clogging. Commonly used ones are no. 4 and no. 5.

Indications

- They maintain a clean surgical field by sucking away blood, secretions, pus, cystic fluids, debris, and flushing solutions.

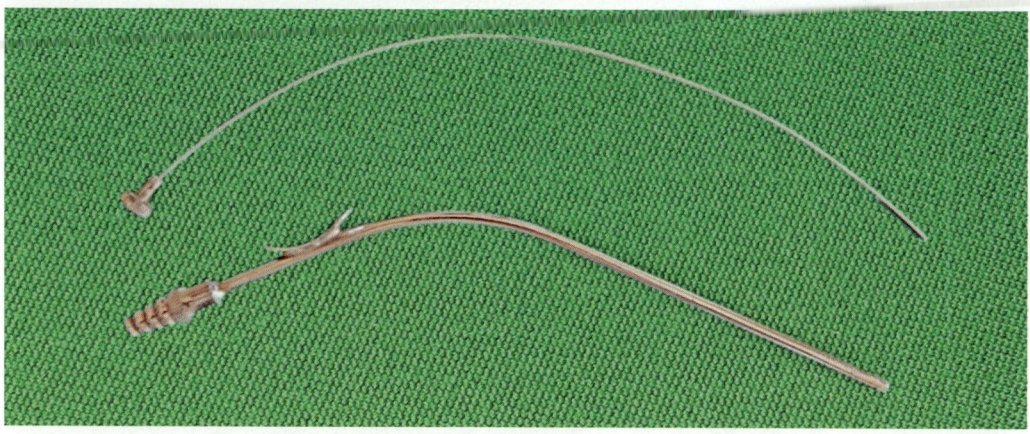

Suction cannula

SYRINGES FOR IRRIGATION

Can be used effectively, and refilled easily with one hand. Difficult to sterilize and large wide bore syringe with 18 gauge needles is needed. Needle should be blunt, smooth and angled for efficient direction of irrigating stream.

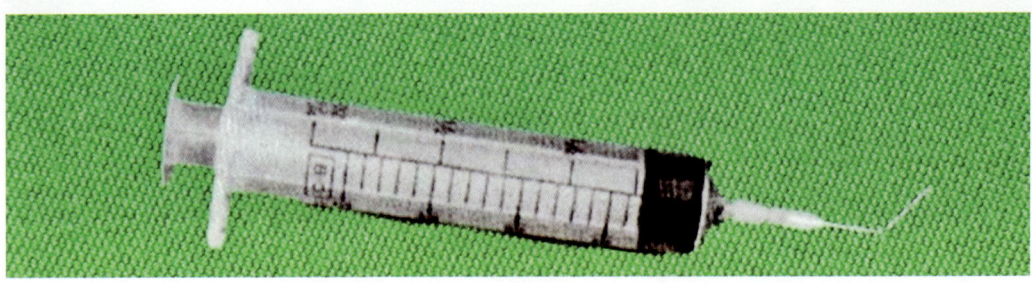

Irrigation syringe

Indication

- Irrigation of surgical field and prevent the heating of bone while bone reduction.

TRIMMING AND FINISHING

BONE RONGUER AND BONE NIBBLERS:

Types

  i. Side cutting
 ii. Side cutting and end cutting

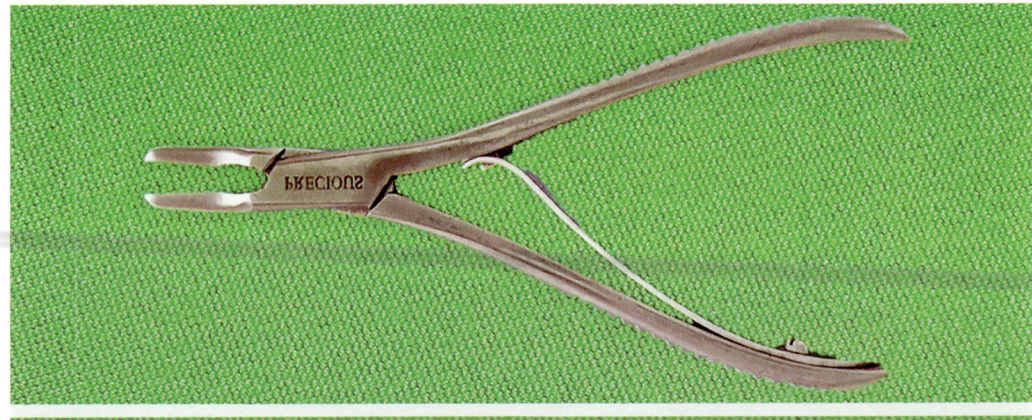

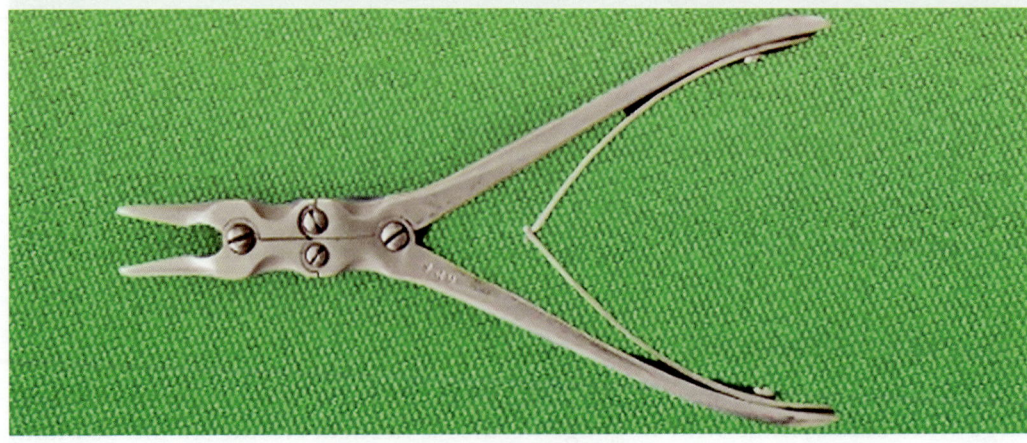

Bone ronguer/bone nibbler

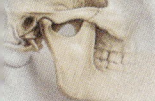

Parts
  i. Beaks
 ii. Hinge joint
iii. Handle with leaf spring.

- Double spring **(Jensen type)** and one spring **(Blumenthal type).**
  It has sharp blades which are squeezed together that causes cutting and pinching action on bone. Leaf spring between the handle leads to opening of the beaks, when pressure is released, it allows repeated cut without manually reopening the beaks.
- **Blumenthal ronguer**
- It is used in dentoalveolar surgical procedures by inserting beaks into socket to cut interradicular bone.
- **Double action nibbler**
  - It cuts the large amount of bone quickly and efficiently.

Indications
- To remove a large amount of bone at a time using multiple, small bites.
- To nibble sharp bony margins following simple or surgical extraction of teeth, surgical procedure alveoloplasty (trim sharp bony ridge).
- To peel off thinned out bone present over cystic, tumorous pathology.

BONE FILE
Parts
  i. Working end
 ii. Shank
iii. Handle.

   It has a working end with different shapes like spherical, oval and curved "c" shape with horizontal serrations used to remove bone by "pull stroke" unidirectionally. It should not be used in push stroke as it causes burning and crushing the bone.

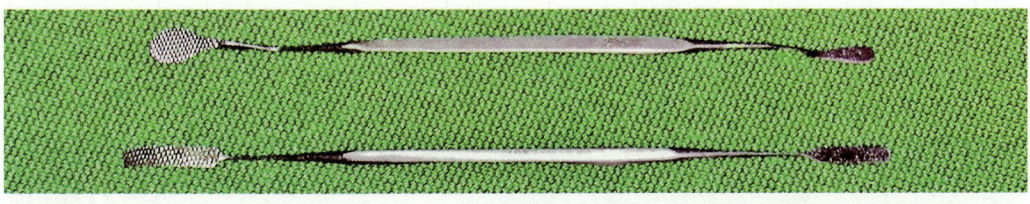

Bone file

Indication
- It is used for final smoothening of bone before suturing of the flap.

MOUTH GAGS

MOUTH PROPS
It consists of vertical block having a concave surface on either of its ends to fit the maxillary and mandibular teeth.

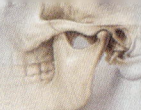

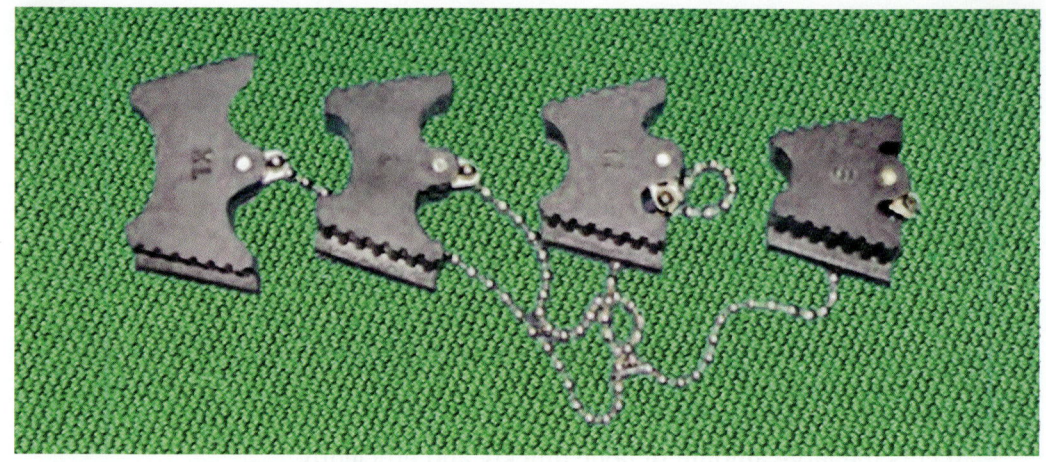

Mouth props

Mouth Props of Various Sizes

Three or four blocks of varying vertical heights are connected by a chain. The operator can choose the block according to the required extent of the oral opening by placing the block in the posterior part of the mouth while the patients bite on it.

Indication

- To hold the patient's mouth open during dental procedures under local and general anesthesia

HEISTER'S JAW OPENER

It has two flat blades with serrations that are applied between the maxillary and mandibular posterior teeth. The two blades are separated by turning key that is positioned between the two blades.

Indication

- To keep the mouth open during oral surgical procedures under local and general anesthesia. For physiotherapy after TMJ ankylosis surgery, oral submucous fibrosis surgery.

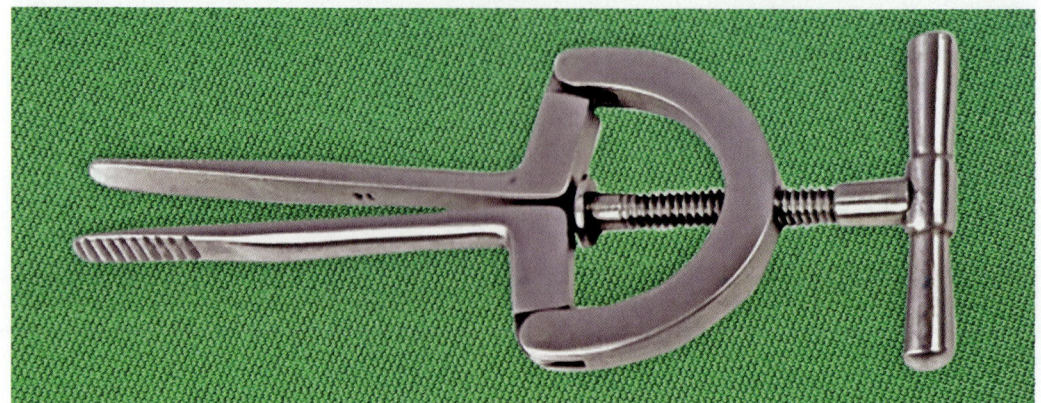

Heister's jaw opener

DOYEN'S MOUTH GAG

It has two C-shaped blades which bear flat extensions at an angle. These extensions have serrations on them that rest on the occlusal surface of teeth. The blades are connected by a joint that is in turn connected to handles similar to that of scissors. The handle has a catch that is fixed at the required opening.

Indication

- It helps to keep the mouth of the patient open during surgical procedures.

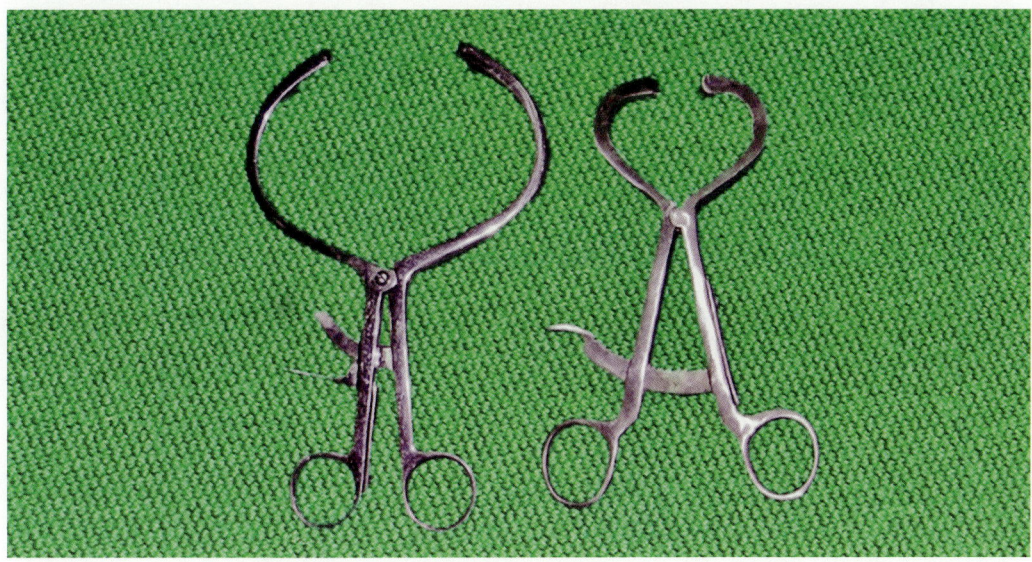

Doyen's mouth gag

FERGUSON'S MOUTH GAG

The Ferguson's mouth gag has two flat blades on the working end with serrations that rest on the occlusal surfaces of maxillary and mandibular teeth.

Blades are not parallel; they are divergent to adapt itself to the divergence of jaw in open position. The handle has a catch that is fixed at the required opening.

Indication

- It helps to keep the mouth of the patient open during the surgical procedures.

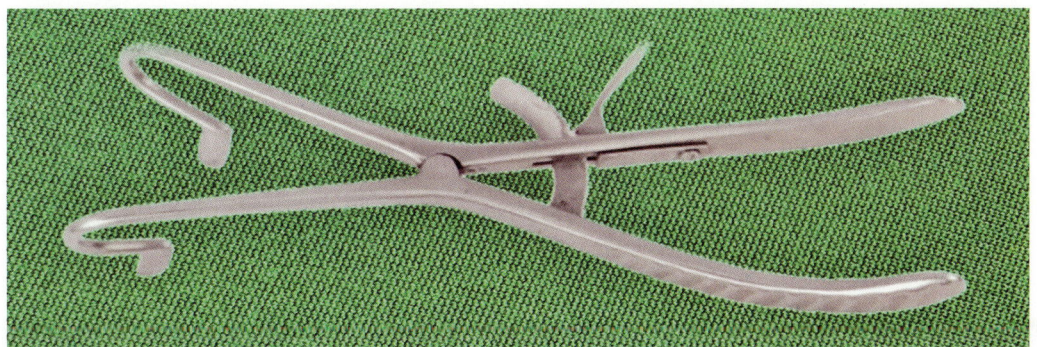

Ferguson's mouth gag

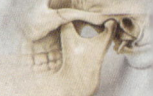

HEMOSTAT

Note: Detailed description in chapter on General Surgery Instruments

SUTURING INSTRUMENTS

- Needle holder.
- Adson's tissue forceps.
- Dean's sutures cutting scissors.

Note: Detailed description of suturing instruments is given in chapter of general surgical instrument.

Maxillofacial Trauma Instrument

M Veerabhau, Paul V Joseph, Shobna

INSTRUMENTS FOR INCISION

SCALPEL

Note: Detailed description in chapter on Minor Oral Surgical Instruments.

ELECTROCAUTERY

Monopolar Electrocautery

1. High frequency AC generator (20000 Hz)
2. Regulator (controls intensity)
3. Foot control

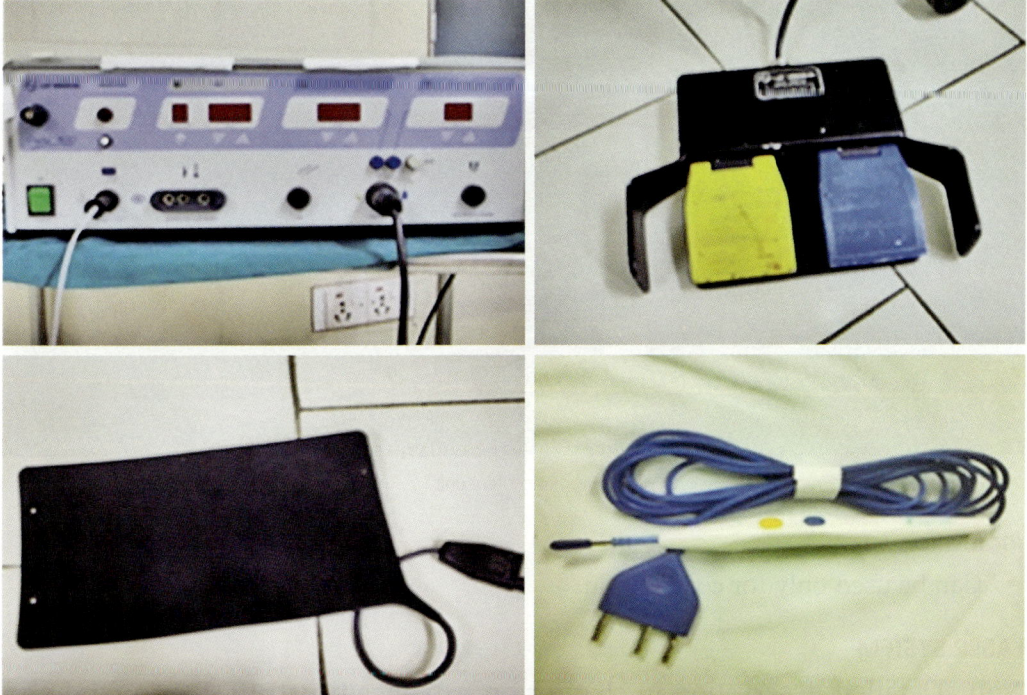

Electrocautery: Monopolar unit

4. Indifferent electrode (acts as earth)
5. Active electrode (a fine tip).

Principle

- The large, flat steel plate or the indifferent electrode acts as the earth.
- Due to large difference between the size of two electrodes, a high current density is generated around the active electrode, resulting in a heating effect.

Precautions

- Care must be taken to ensure intimate contact between patient and indifferent electrode, usually by a wet cloth wrapped on an electrode.
- Avoid placement of indifferent electrode near bony ridges.
- Do not use near nerves and isolated vascular pedicles.
- Operator should wear rubber footwear.
- Risk of sparking is high with ether or cyclopropane (used as general anesthetics).

Indications

- Coagulation of small bleeders and cutting of soft tissues.
- Fulguration (burns the tissue margins, useful in resecting small growths).

Bipolar Cautery Unit

- No indifferent electrode.
- AC is low power.
- Active electrode is the form of forceps as it has two ends (two electrodes).

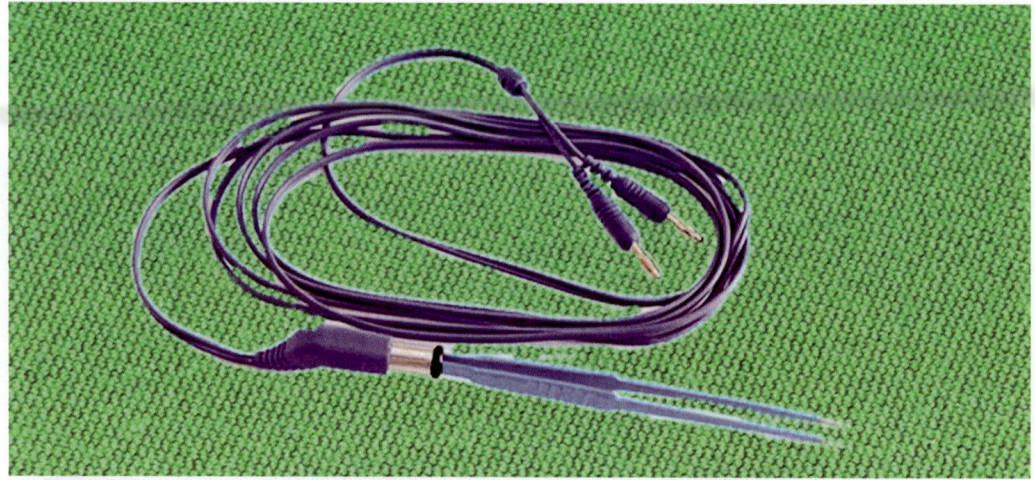

Bipolar cautery unit

Indication

- Can be used only for coagulation.

LASER SYSTEM

Note: Detailed description in chapter on Advanced Instruments in Oral and Maxillofacial Surgery.

DISSECTING SCISSORS

Used to perform soft tissue dissection in deeper layers. Can be—straight or curved; sharp (Iris, Dean) or blunt (Metzenbaum, Mayo). Curved scissors are more preferred by the surgeons for dissecting as they provide better vision of the operating area. The tips of scissors are also used to spread and probe the area of incision. Smaller sizes are used at surface, the larger sizes used deeper in cavities.

Indication

- It is used to dissect different tissue planes during surgical operations and to cut or divide important structures.

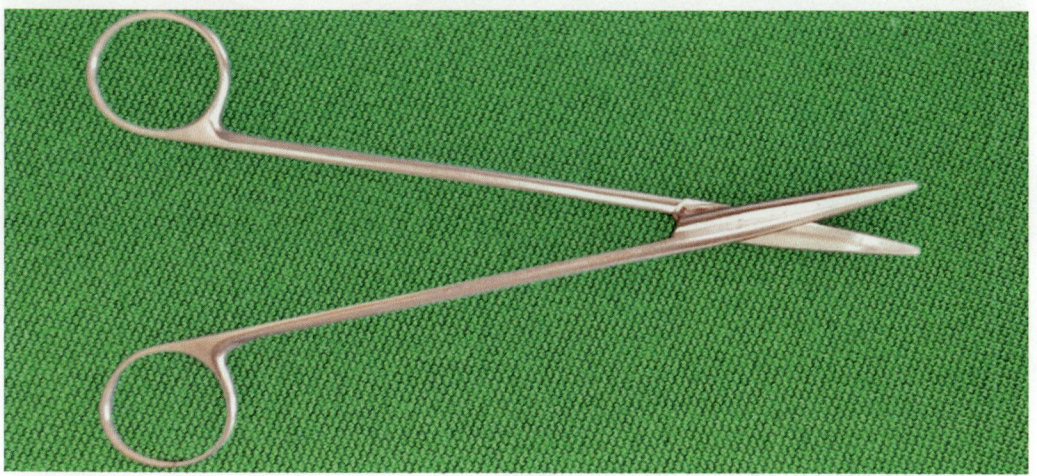

Dissecting scissors

METZENBAUM SCISSORS

Longer, blunt nosed, larger handle to blade ratio.

Indication

- For undermining the tissue.

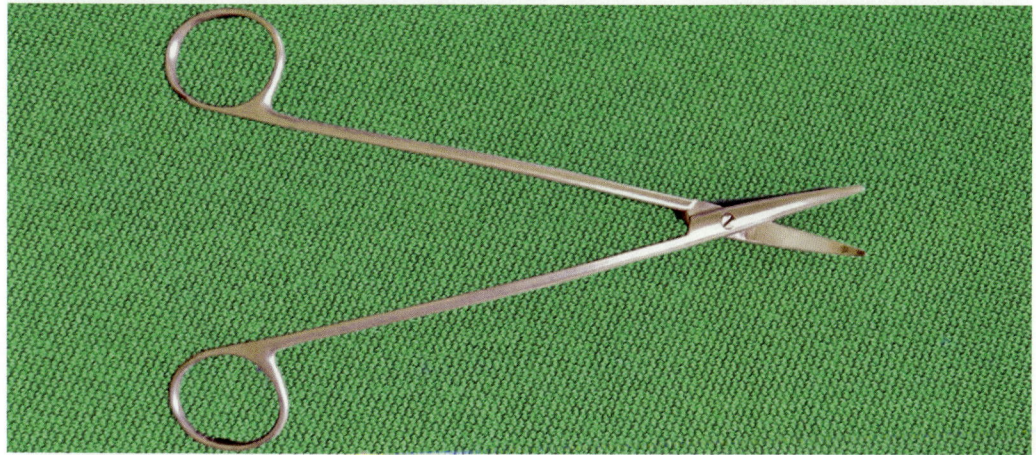

Metzenbaum scissors

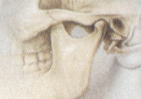

MAYO SCISSORS

These scissors are heavier compared to Metzenbaum scissors.

Indication

- Cutting heavy fascia (curved) and sutures (straight).

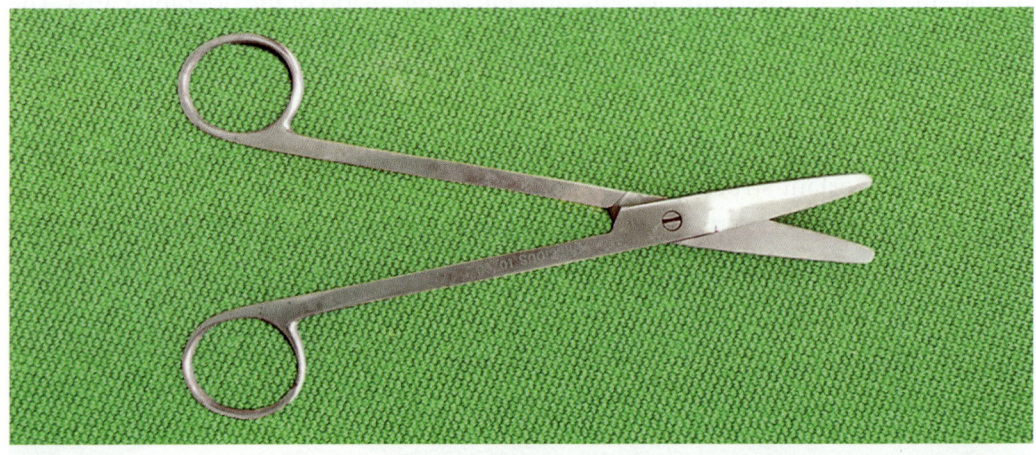

Mayo scissors

IRIS SCISSORS

Small, sharp, pointed, delicate with curved or angular cutting blades (for fine work).

Indication

- They are used to remove necrotic tissue.

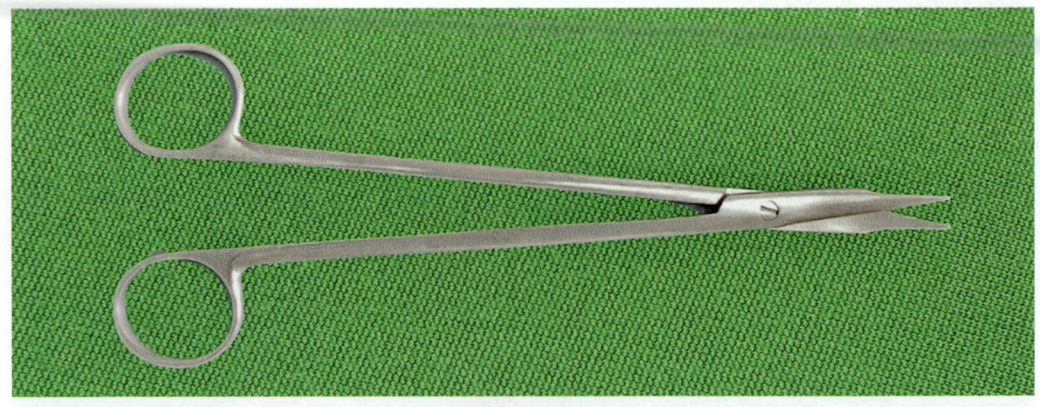

Iris scissors

MOSQUITO FORCEPS

Note: Detailed description in chapter on General Surgical Instruments.

SKIN HOOK

Note: Detailed description in chapter on General Surgical Instruments.

INSTRUMENTS FOR REFLECTION

PERIOSTEAL ELEVATOR

Note: Detailed description in chapter on Minor Oral Surgical Instruments.

PERIOSTEAL STRIPPER

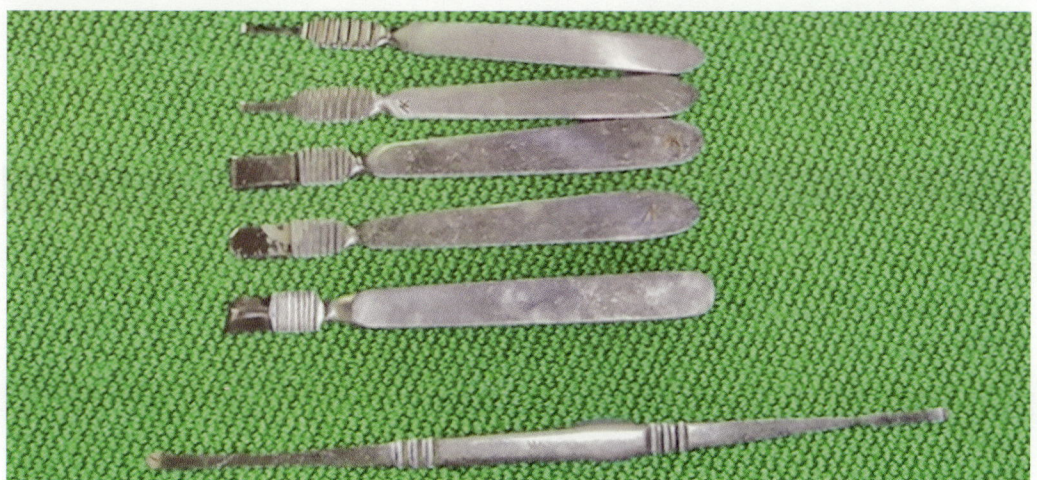

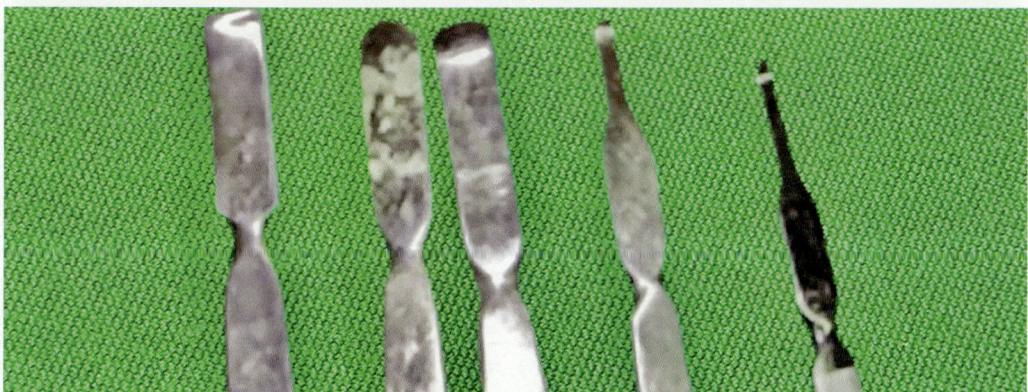

Periosteal stripper

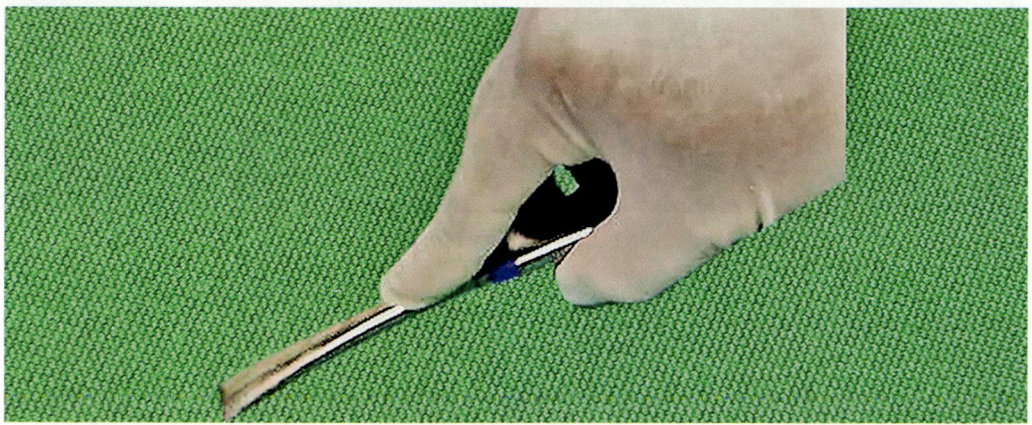

How to use?

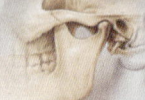

How to Use?

Light in weight. Used in "push" stroke.

Indication

It is used to elevate periosteum in quicker and easier fashion.

HOWARTH'S ELEVATOR

Note: Detailed description in chapter on Minor Oral Surgical Instruments.

INSTRUMENTS FOR RETRACTION

Self-retaining Retractors

SELF-RETAINING MASTOID RETRACTOR

Indication

- It is used to provide good vision and good access to perform surgery in the mastoid region.

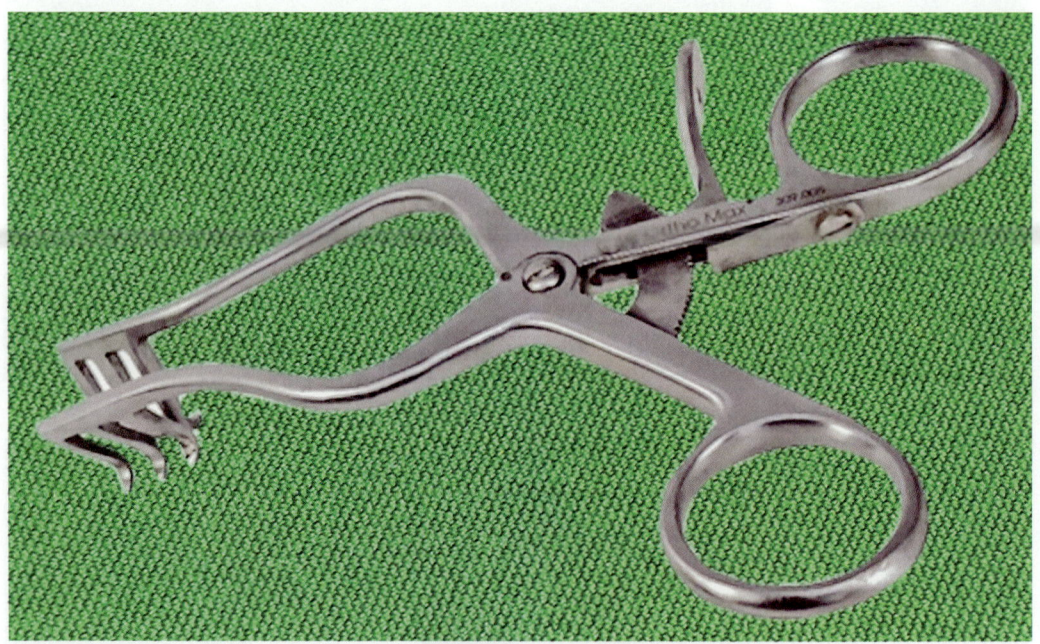

Self-retaining mastoid retractor

SELF-RETAINING SKIN RETRACTOR

Indication

- It is used for retracting skin to provide good vision and good access to perform surgery.

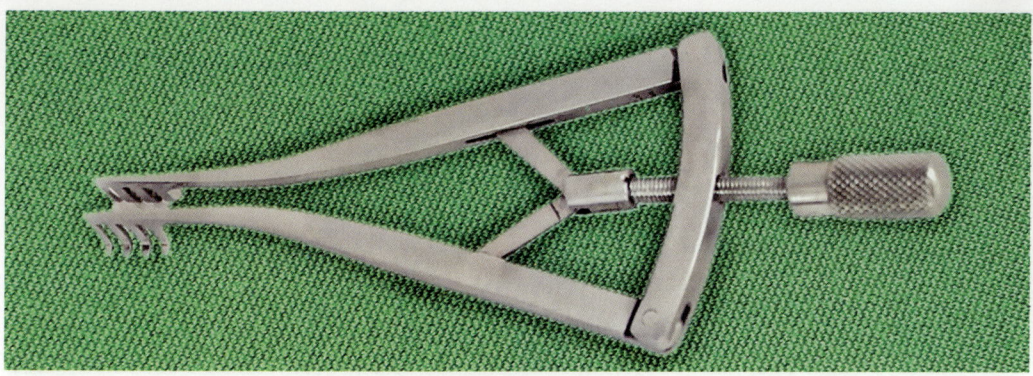

Self-retaining skin retractor

Plain and Hand Held Retractors

LANGENBACK RETRACTOR

Note: Detailed description in chapter on General Surgical Instruments.

ORBITAL FLOOR RETRACTOR

It has a broad handle and a connecting slender shank with an offset having a flat broad quadrangular working end.

Indication

- It is used for the retraction of the orbital contents from the orbital floor during the reconstruction of the floor of the orbit.

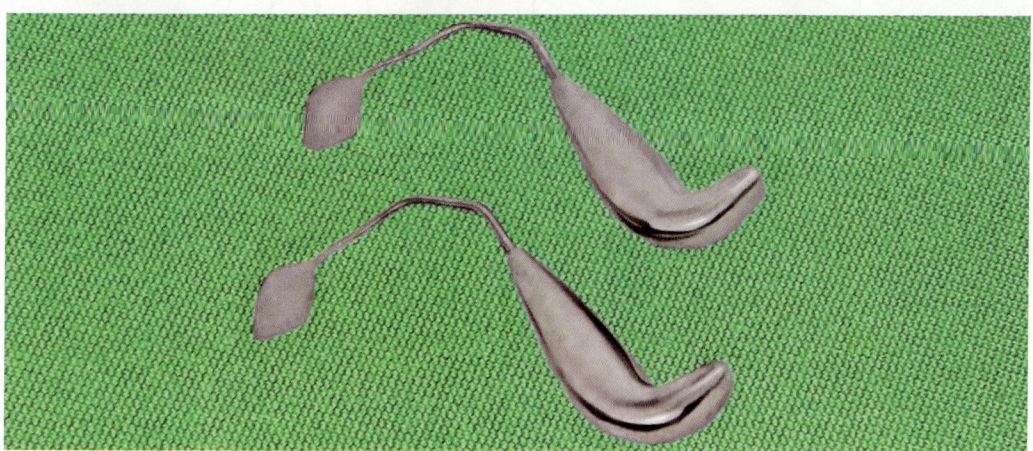

Orbital floor retractor

OBWEGESSOR'S RAMUS RETRACTORS

Indications

- To retract soft tissue along the anterior border of the ramus during sagittal split ramus osteotomy.
- Ramus retractors are used to retract the tissue over the anterior aspect of the ascending ramus of the mandible in surgery involving this area.
- To retract the tissues during coronoidectomy.
- To retract soft tissue over the anterior nasal spine during Le-fort I osteotomy.

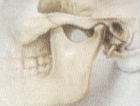

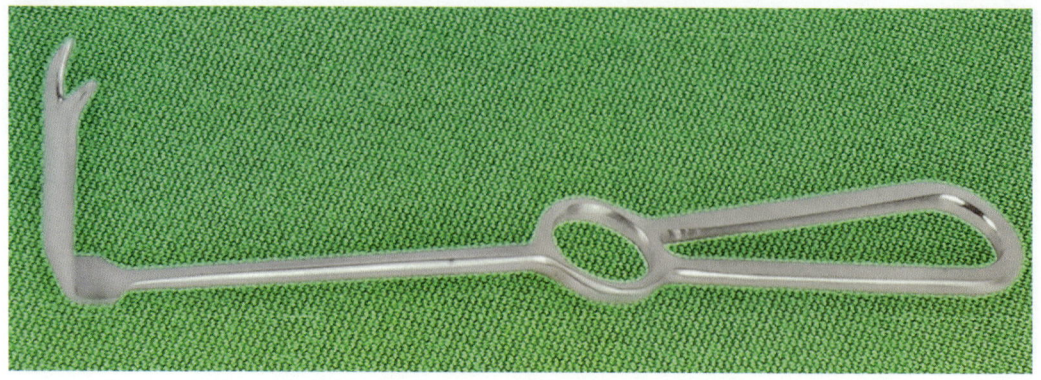

Obwegessor's ramus retractors

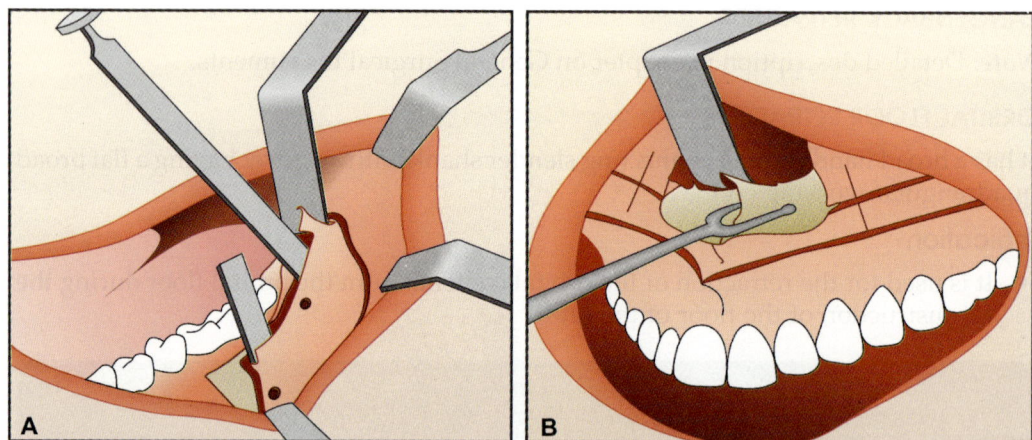

How to use?

CONDYLE RETRACTOR

Indications

*   It is used to retract the soft tissue in condylar region.
*   'C' shaped tip is slipped under the ankylosed mass to retract and protect the medial soft tissue during TMJ surgery.

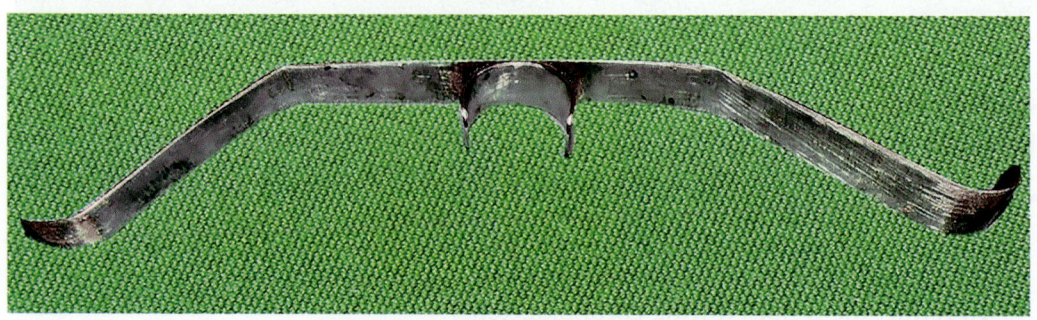

Condyle retractor

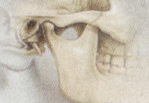

CHIN RETRACTOR

Indication

- Chin retractor is used for retracting chin in case of genioplasty, chin reduction and other procedures involving chin.

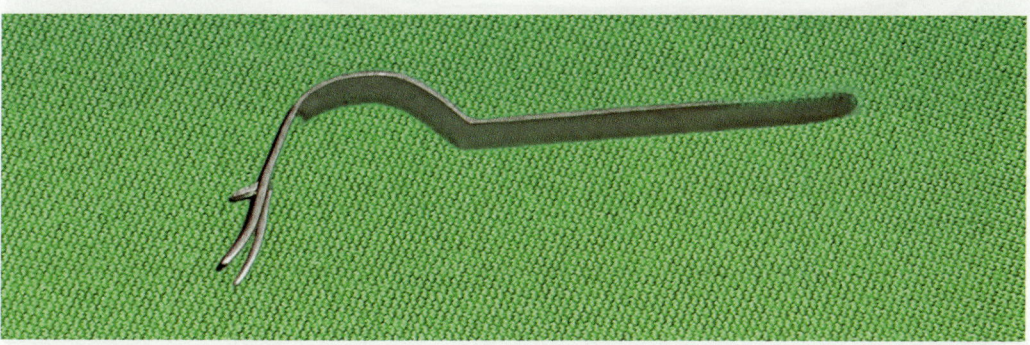

Chin retractor

CHANNEL RETRACTOR

Indications

- Narrow channel retractor is used for placement on the lingual aspect of the mandible.
- The wider channel retractor is used to engage the inferior border of the mandible on the facial side to assist in this portion of osteotomy.

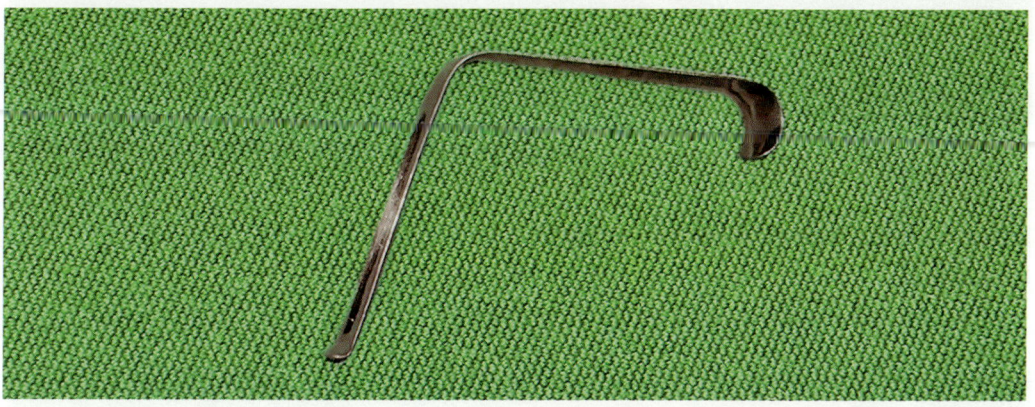

Channel retractor

MANDIBULAR BODY RETRACTOR

Indication

- The mandibular body retractor cradles the inferior border of the mandible to:
  - Facilitate making the vertical cut of the midsagittal osteotomy.
  - Distend the cheek.
  - Protect the facial artery and vein.
  - Support the mandible as the osteotomes are struck with a mallet.
  - Permit an adequate cut of the inferior border.

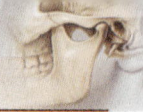

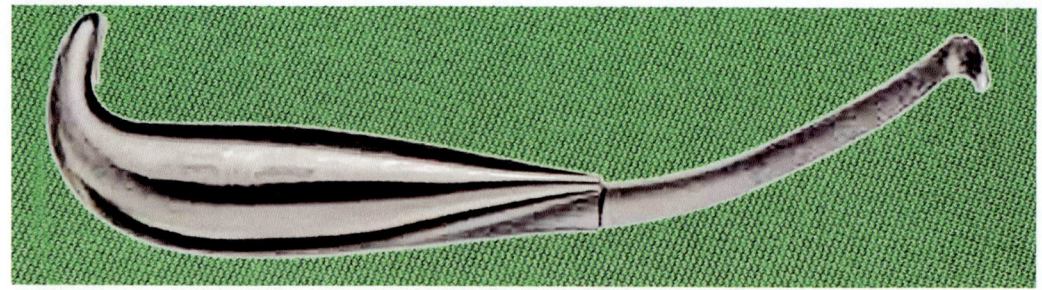

Mandibular body retractor

SIGMOID NOTCH RETRACTOR

Indication

- It is used to retract the sigmoid notch in maxillofacial trauma in ramus and condyle region.

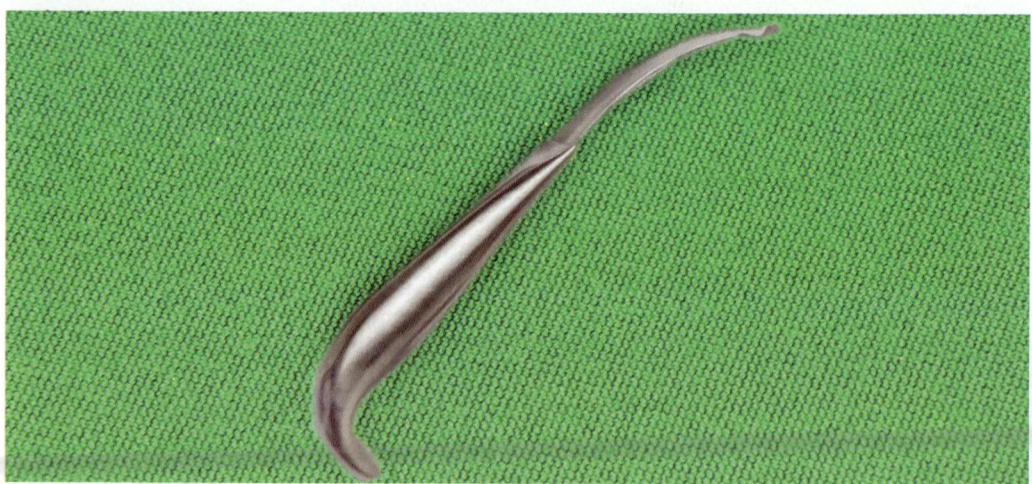

Sigmoid notch retractor

DOYEN'S RASPATORY (RIB RETRACTOR)

Indication

- To elevate the inner periosteum of a rib during the rib resection for harvesting the rib.

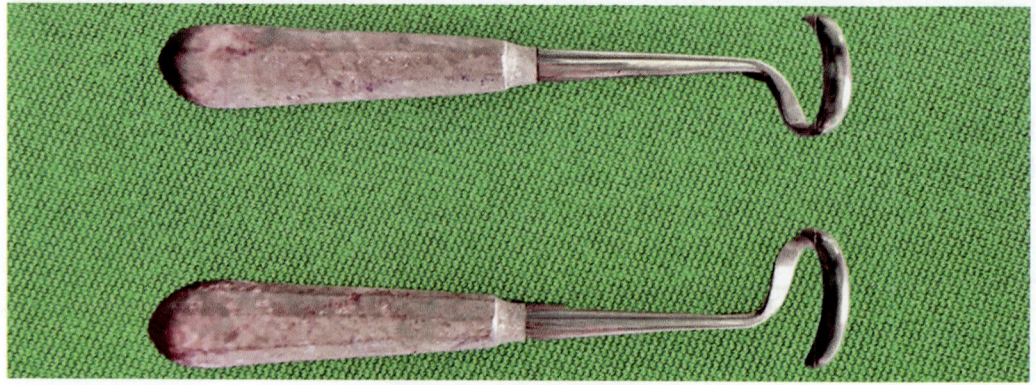

Doyen's raspatory (rib retractor)

TONGUE DEPRESSOR
Indications
- To retract tongue during surgery in oral cavity.
- For inspection of oral cavity, tonsils and pharyngeal wall.

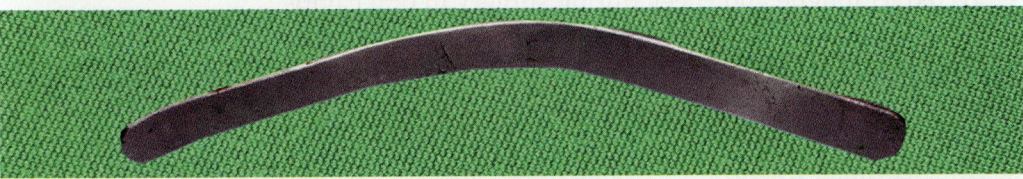

Tongue depressor

WEIDER TONGUE RETRACTOR
Indication
- To depress the tongue during endotracheal intubation and extubation.

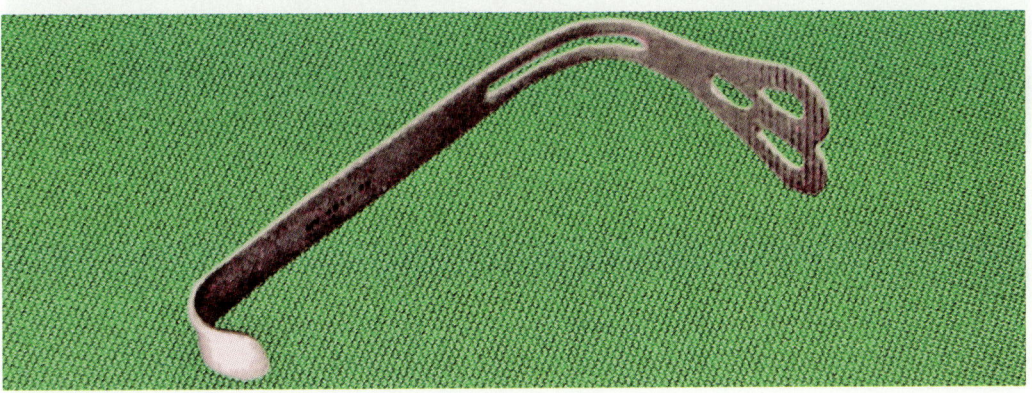

Weider tongue retractor

C-SHAPED RETRACTOR (DEAVER'S RETRACTOR)
Indication
- It is used to retract soft tissues like cheek. Mostly used in abdominal surgeries.

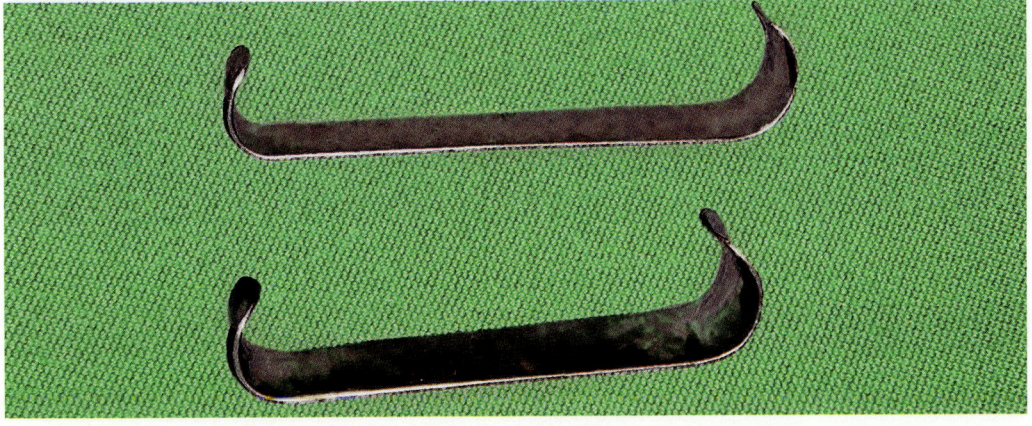

C-shaped retractor (Deaver's retractor)

UNIVERSAL RETRACTOR

Indications

- To depress the tongue during endotracheal intubation and extubation.
- For inspection of oral cavity, tonsils and pharyngeal wall.
- To retract tongue and cheek during surgery in oral cavity.

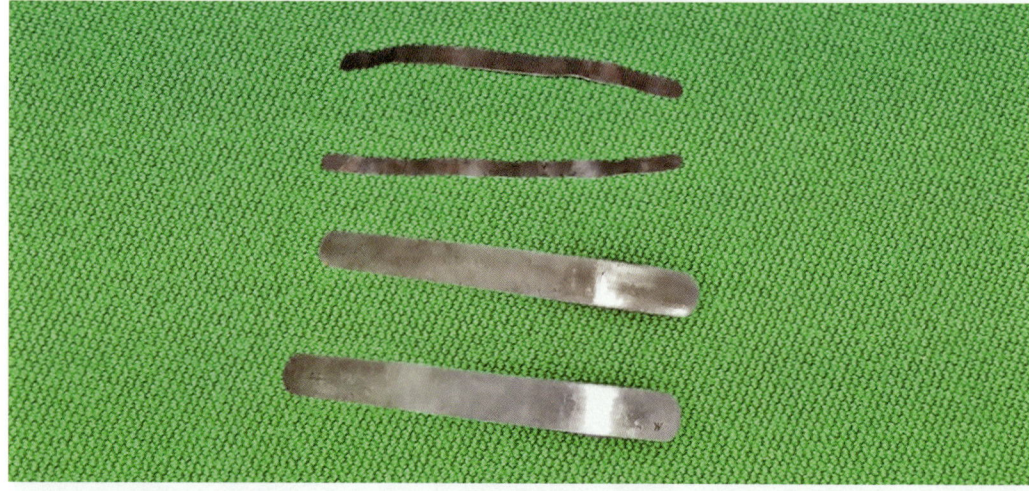

Universal retractor

NERVE HOOK (DANDY'S)

Indication

- Used in neurectomy procedures for nerve identification and in nerve repositioning procedures.

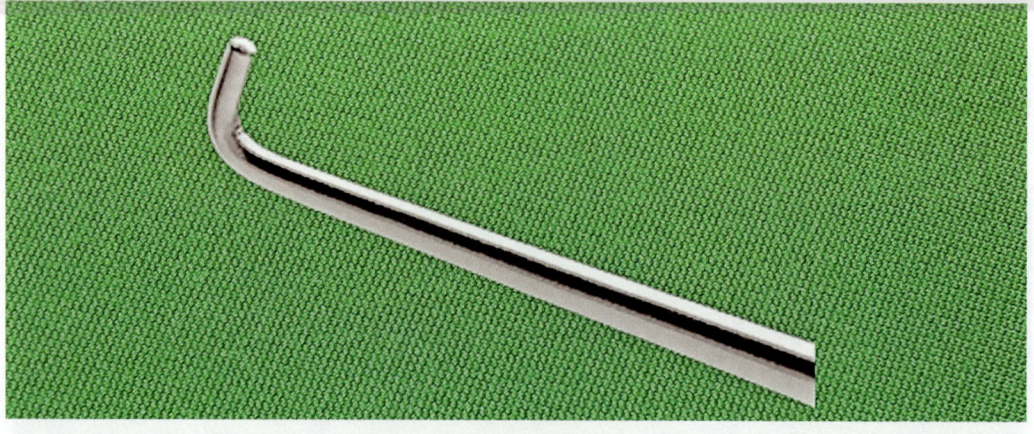

Nerve hook (Dandy's)

INSTRUMENTS FOR CURETTAGE

Soft tissue curettes

Note: Detailed description in chapter on Minor Oral Surgical Instruments.

INSTRUMENTS FOR REDUCTION

FERGUSSON'S LION JAW BONE HOLDING FORCEPS
Indications

- Use to hold bone during open reduction of a fracture.
- Use to hold maxilla/mandible during maxillectomy/mandibulectomy, respectively.

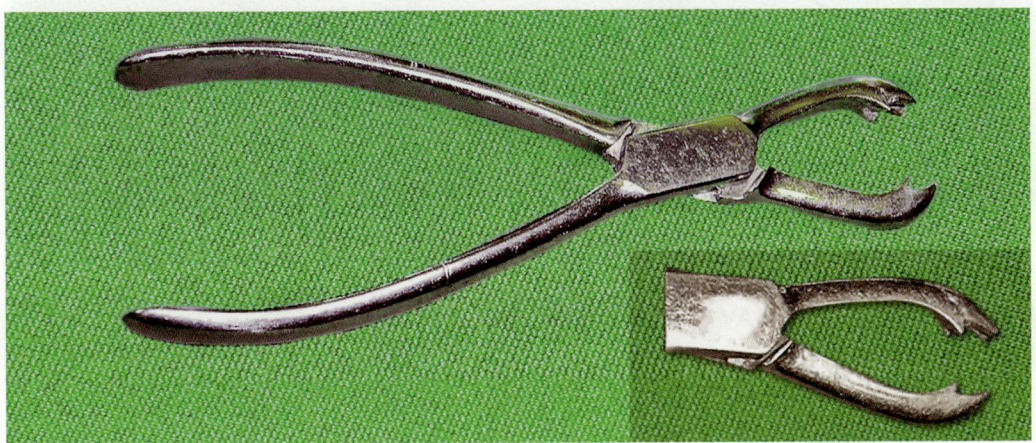

Fergusson's lion jaw bone holding forceps

ROWE'S BONE HOLDING FORCEPS
Indication

- It is used to hold bone during open reduction of a fracture of mandible.

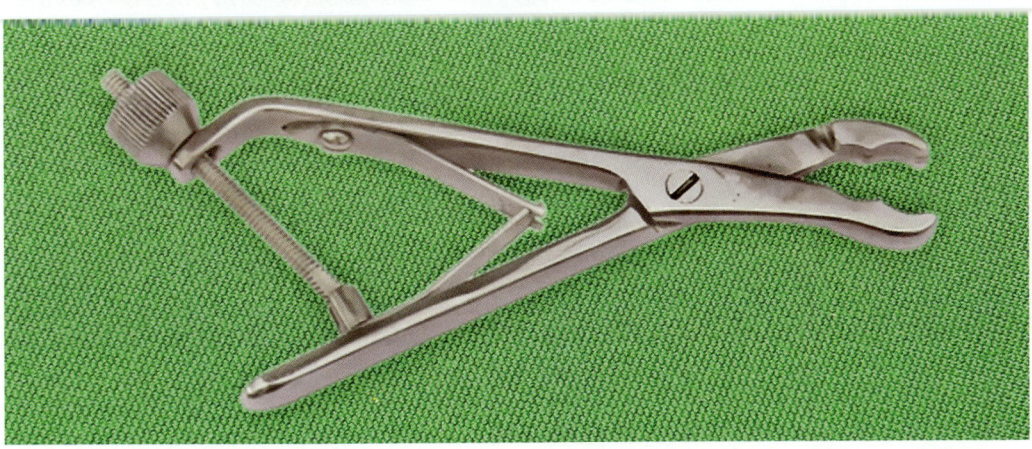

Rowe's bone holding forceps

BONE REDUCTION FORCEPS
Indication

- It is used to reduce and hold the fractured segment in anatomic position for proper reduction of bone.

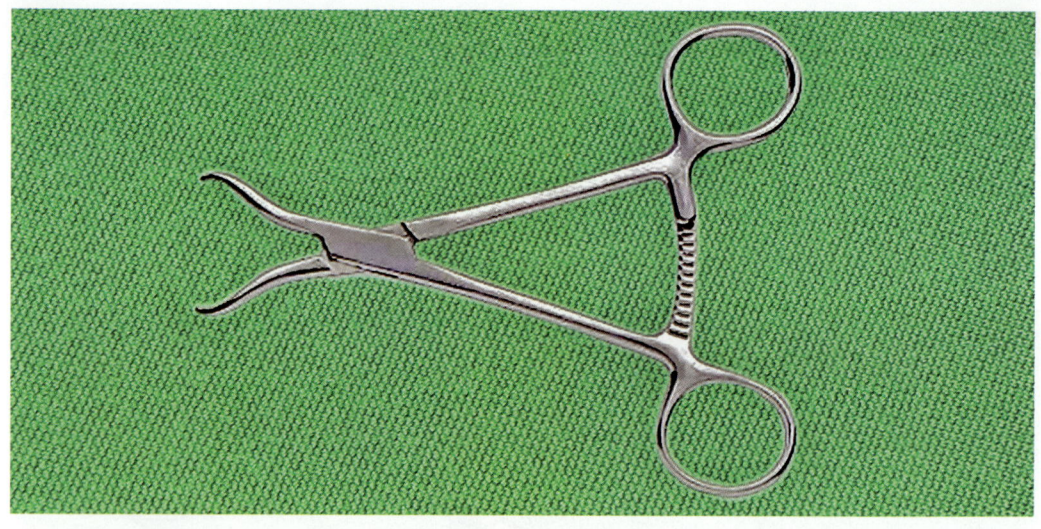

Bone reduction forceps

KOCHER'S TOOTHED HEAVY ARTERY FORCEPS

Indications

- Instrument is specially designed to hold the coronoid process during coronoidectomy.
- For stabilizing the fractured ends.
- To remove a sequestrum from an osteomyelitic lesion.

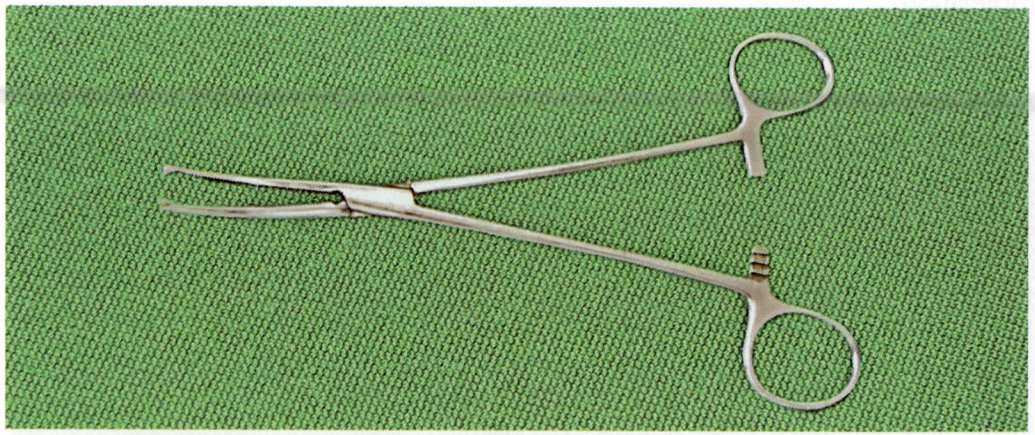

Kocher's toothed heavy artery forceps

ROWE'S MAXILLARY DISIMPACTION FORCEPS

How to Use?

- The operator stands behind the patient and grasps the handles of the forceps and manipulates the fragments into position.
- First traction is in upward direction. Then, it is in downward and forward direction. Finally, it is in forward direction with rocking and rotational movements in both horizontal and vertical axis.

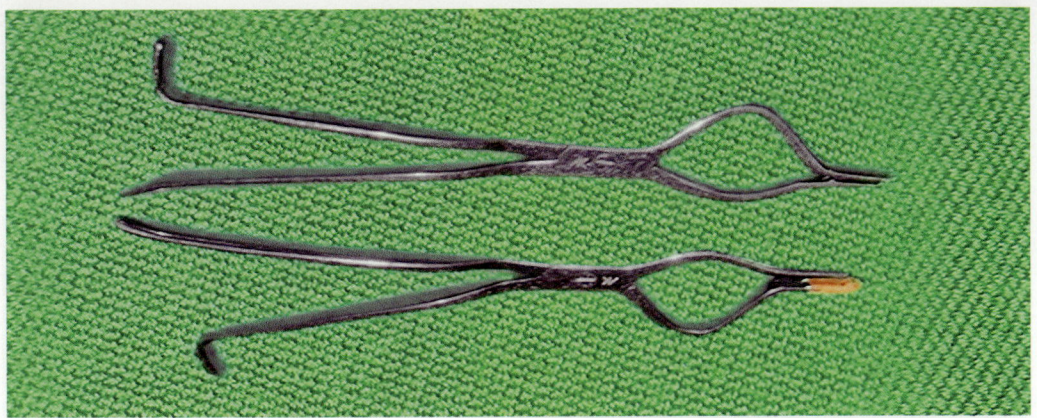

Rowe's maxillary disimpaction forceps

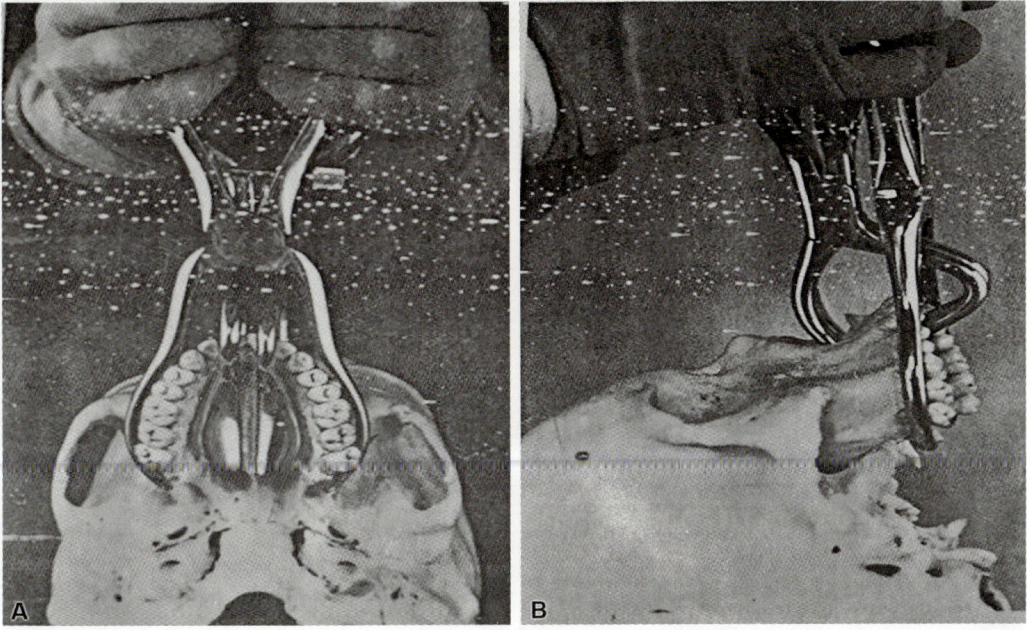

How to use?

Indication

- This instrument is used in pairs for reduction of maxilla in Lefort fractures where the maxilla is impacted.

HAYTON WILLIAM'S FORCEPS
How to Use?

- The inner aspects of both blades are made to fit against the buccal aspect of the alveolus of maxilla.
- Pressure is directed towards the midline via both the blades for approximation of the bones.
- A screw is present at the top to prevent crushing of the bone.

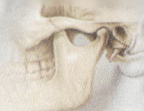

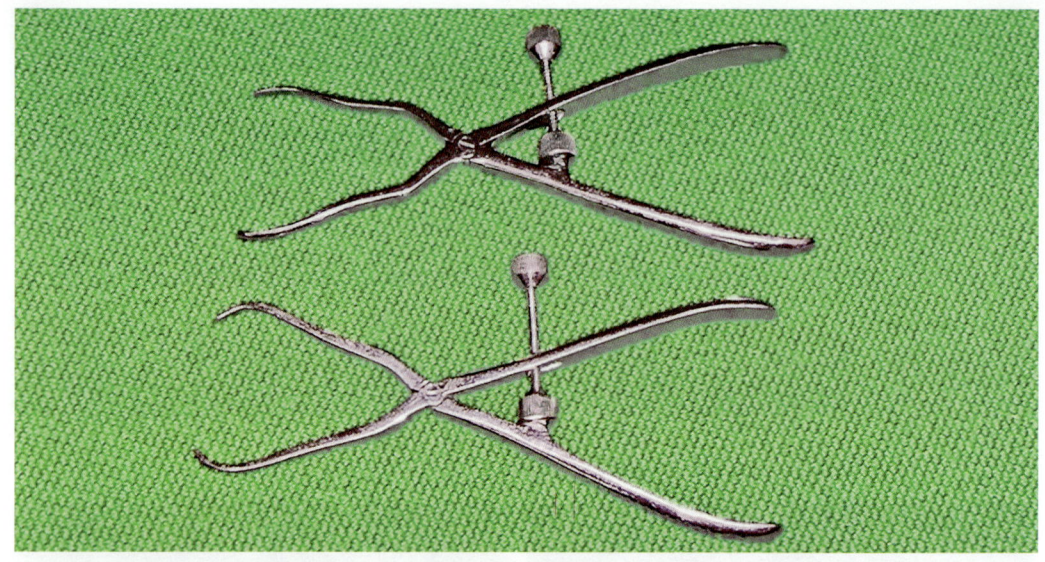

Hayton William's forceps

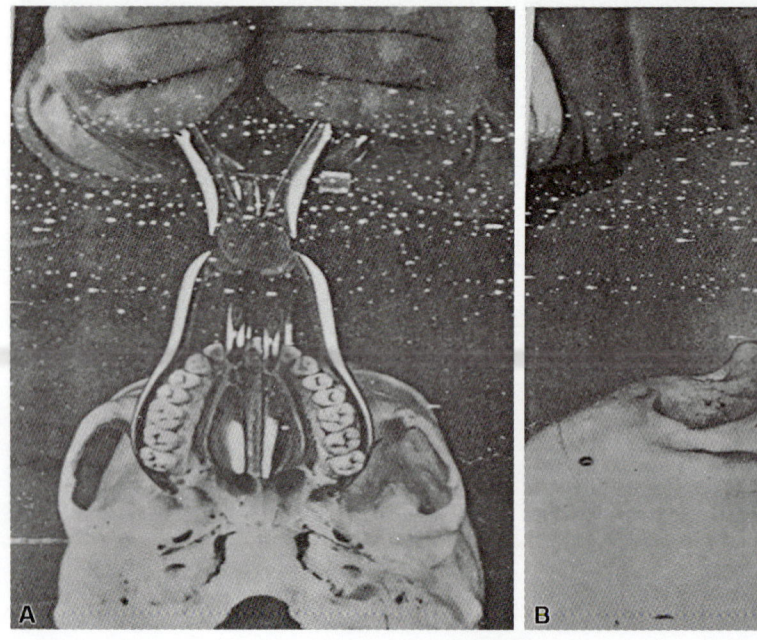

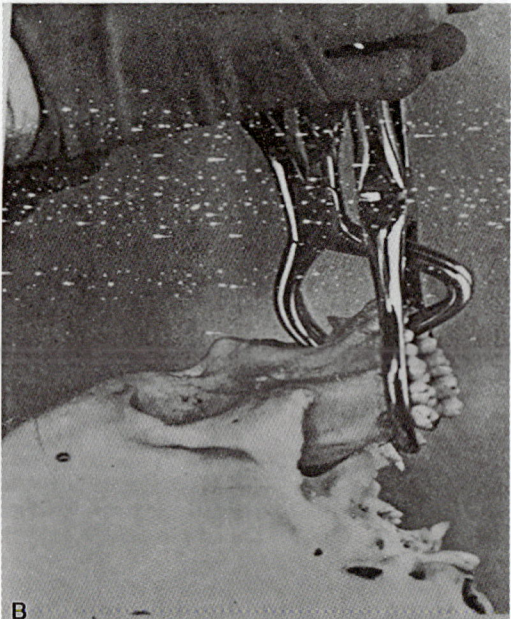

How to Use?

Indication

- It is used to mobilize the maxilla along with Rowe's maxillary disimpaction forceps.

ASCH'S NASAL SEPTAL FORCEPS

How to Use?

- When reducing the nasal septum both the blades are inserted internally, one on each side of the septum.
- In case of nasal bone fracture reduction, one blade is inserted internally and other one is placed externally to hold the nasal bone laterally and medially respectively.

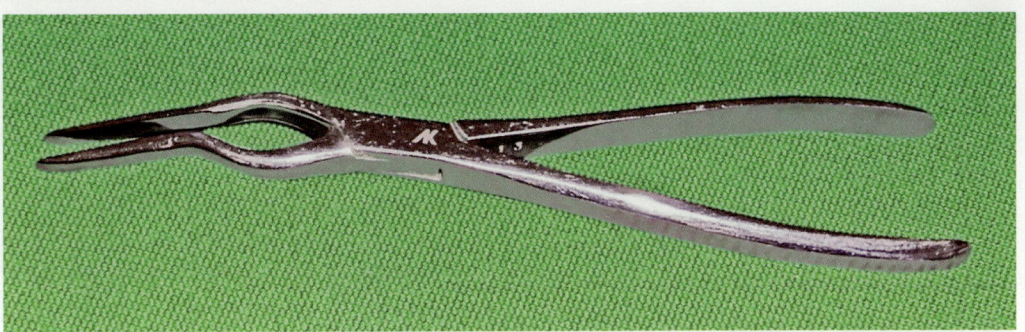

Asch's nasal septal forceps

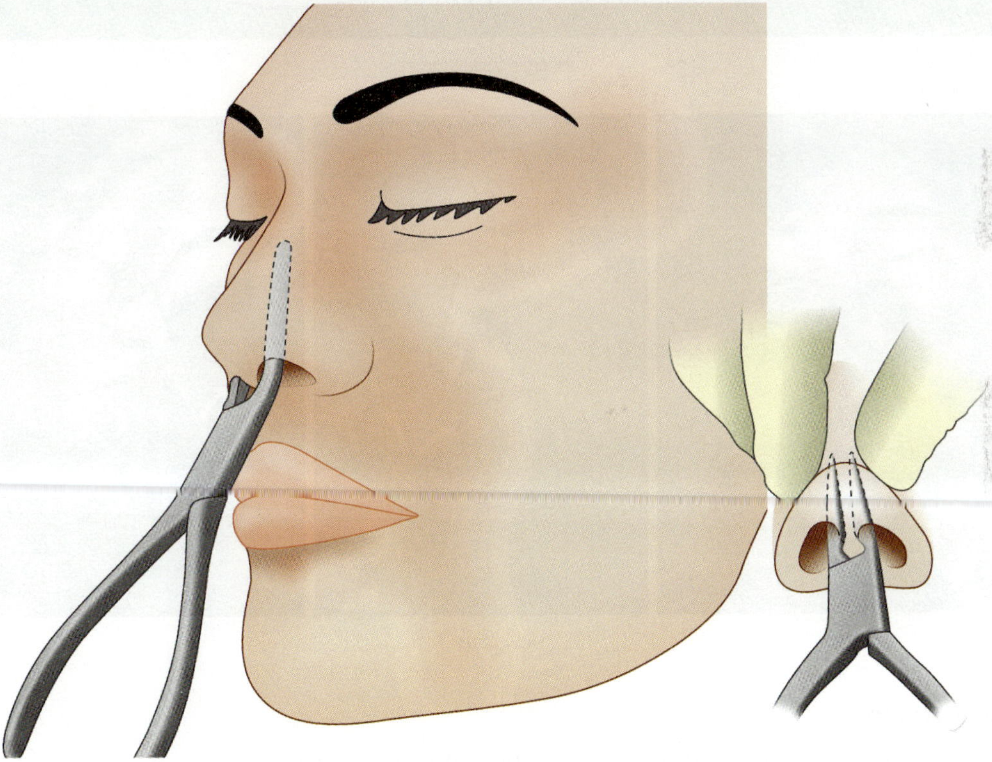

How to use?

Indication

- This instrument is used to reduce the fracture of the nasal bone and to align the nasal septum.

WALSHAM'S SEPTAL FORCEPS
How to Use?

- The padded blade is placed externally into a nostril and the unpadded blade is inserted internally and manipulated for the reduction of the nasal fracture.

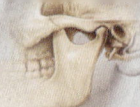

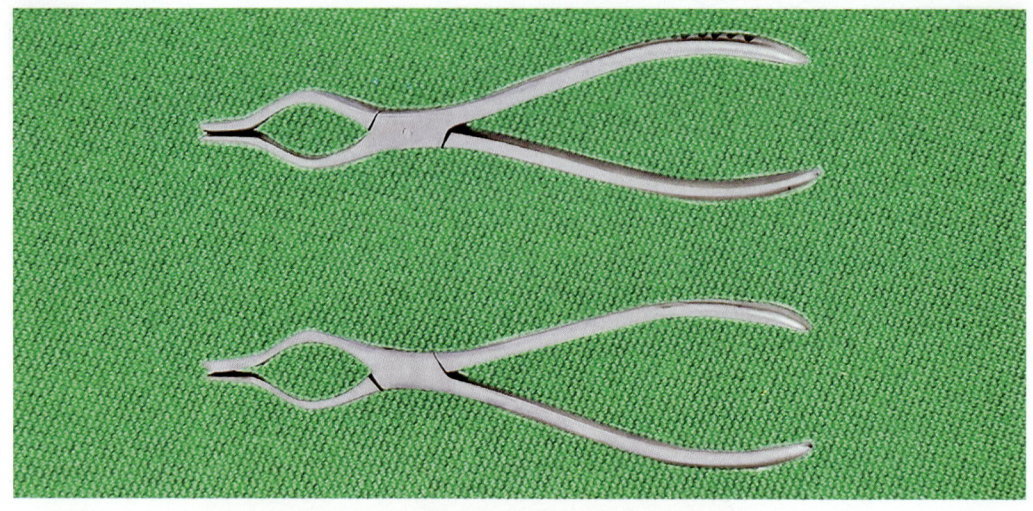

Walsham's septal forceps

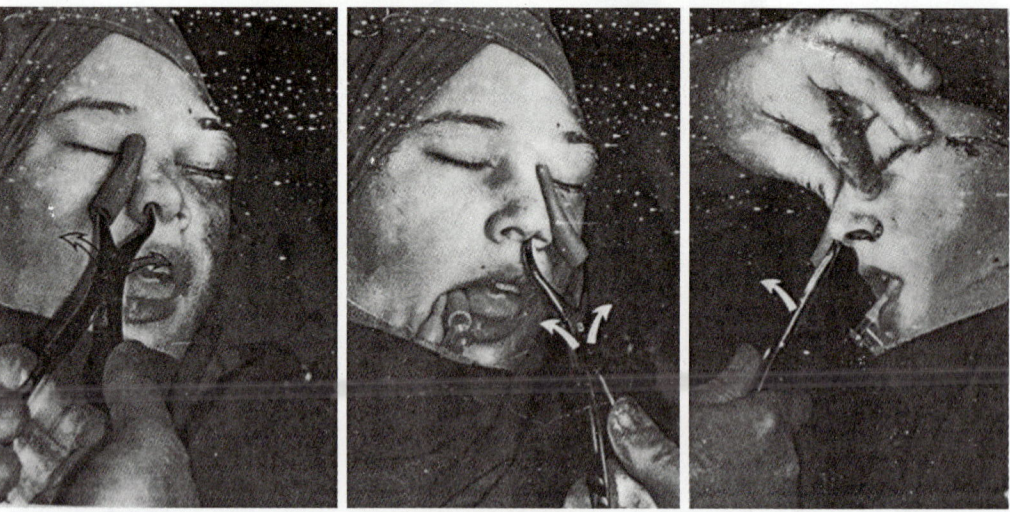

How to use?

Indication

- These forceps are used for the reduction of nasal fracture.

BRISTOW'S ZYGOMA ELEVATOR

How to Use?

- It is passed in between the temporal fascia and temporalis muscle through Gillie's temporal approach.
- The medial aspect of the bone is engaged and elevated to correct the flattening of malar bones and step in lower rim of orbit.

Indication

- This instrument is used to reduce the fractured zygomatic complex and zygomatic arch through the Gillie's temporal approach.

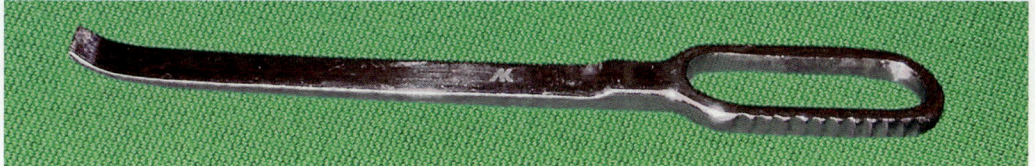

Bristow's zygoma elevator

ROWE'S MODIFICATION OF BRISTOW'S ZYGOMA ELEVATOR

How to Use?

- It is inserted just deep to the depressed zygomatic arch from superior aspect, standing behind the patient through Gillie's temporal approach and an outward force is applied.
- Great care should be taken not to fulcrum off the squamous portion of the temporal bone.

Indication

- This instrument is used to reduce the fractured zygoma through the Gillie's temporal approach.

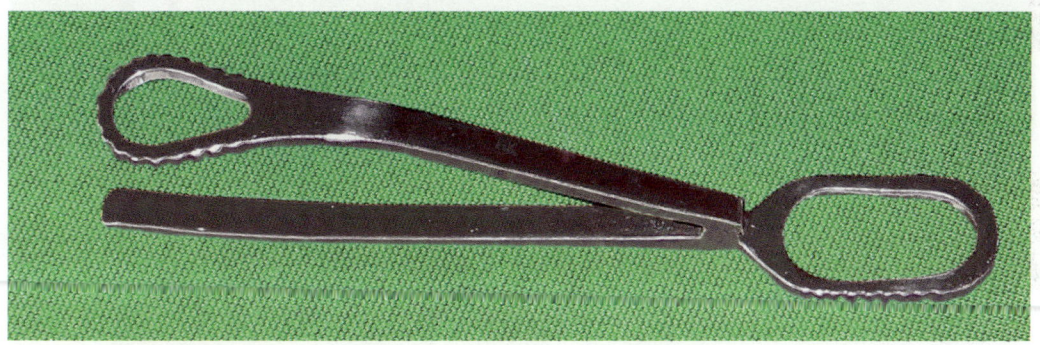

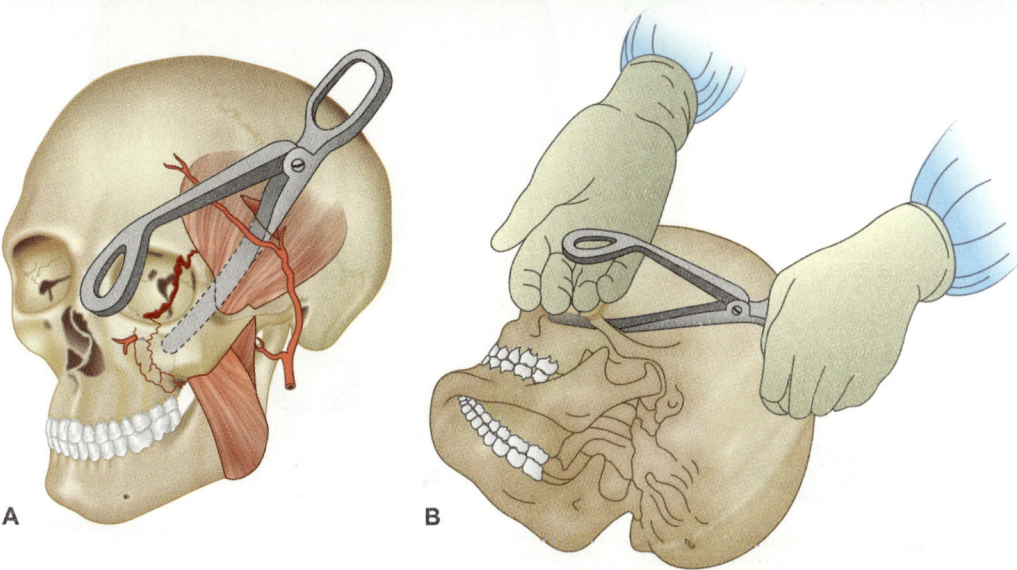

A   B

How to use?

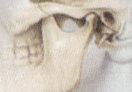

Zygoma Hook (Stacey's pattern)

How to Use?

- It is inserted through the incision below and behind the malar prominence.
- An outward force is applied for proper reduction of the zygoma.

Indication

- This instrument is used to reduce the fractured zygoma through extraoral (percutaneous) stab incision placed at intersection of Poswillo's lines which are drawn from the lateral canthus of eye downwards and from the ala of the nose posteriorly.

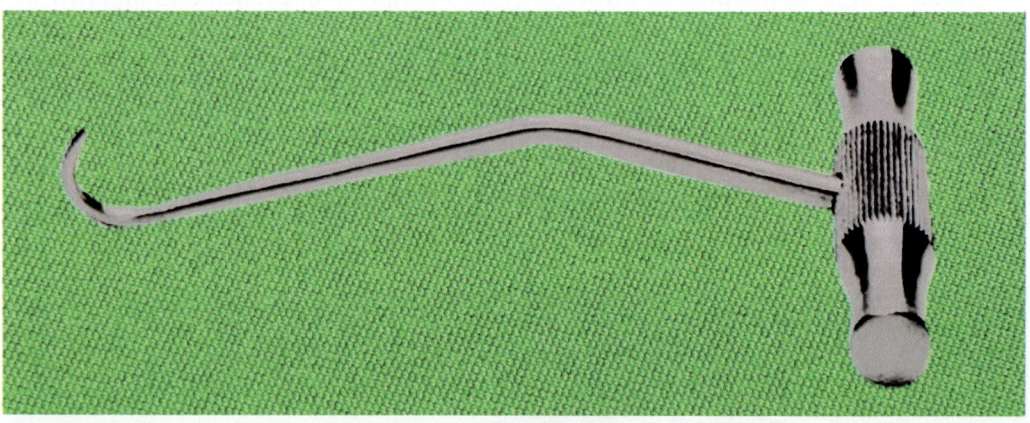

Zygoma hook (Stacey's pattern)

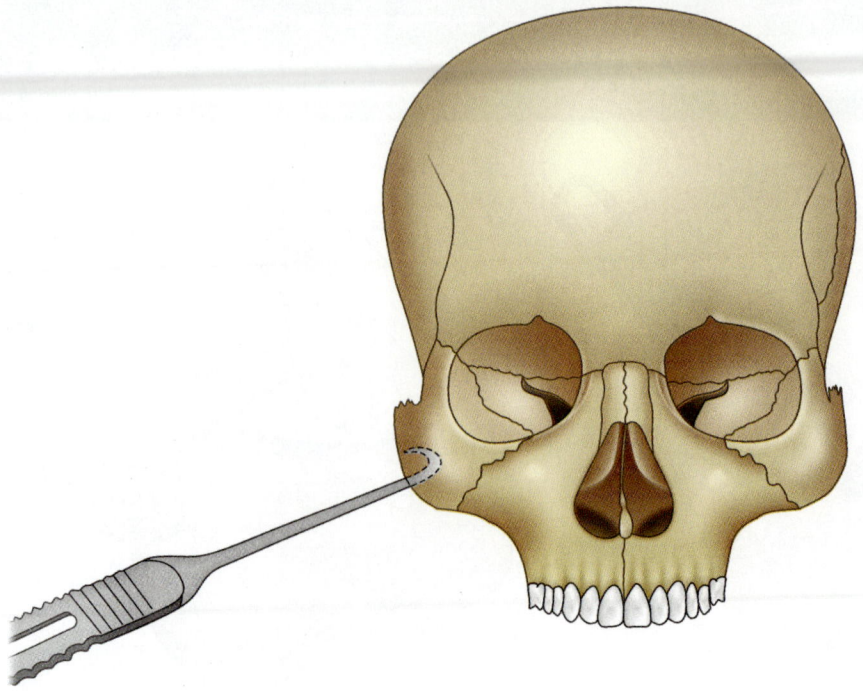

How to use?

BONE AWL (KELSEYFRY'S BONE AWL)

Indications

- It is used for circummandibular and circumzygomatic wiring. Curved bone awl with tip is mostly used.
- It is used for per alveolar wiring.
- It is also used for closed reduction of edentulous mandible with gunning splint
- It is used for holding the reduced fractured fragments in position by means of circumferential wires.

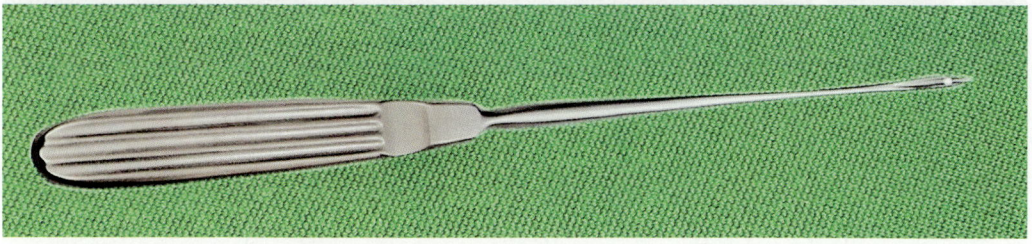

Bone awl (Kelseyfry's bone awl)

INSTRUMENTS FOR OSTEOTOMY

GIGLI'S WIRE SAW AND INTRODUCER

Indications

- When moved to and fro along its long axis, it cuts the bone.
- Used in mandibulectomy procedures.

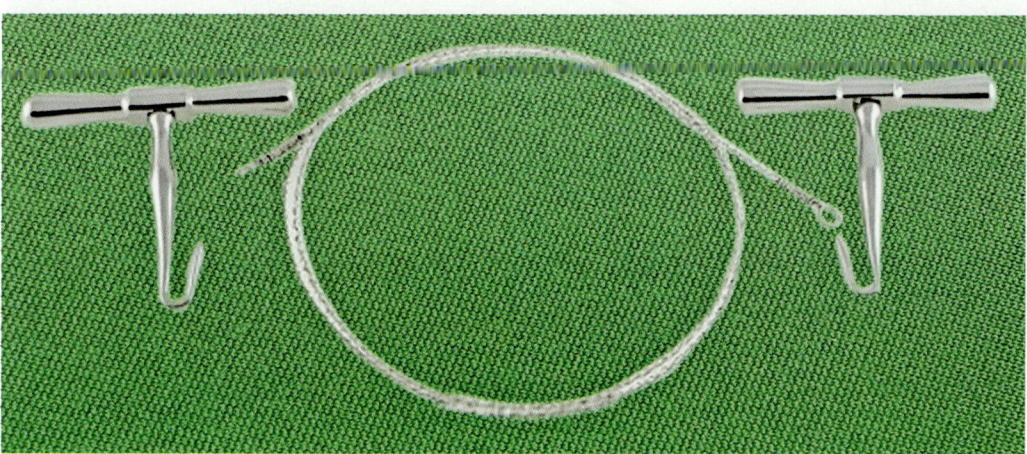

Gigli's wire saw and introducer

OSTEOTOME

Indications

- Various osteotomy procedures in maxillofacial region.
- Removal/recontouring of bone.

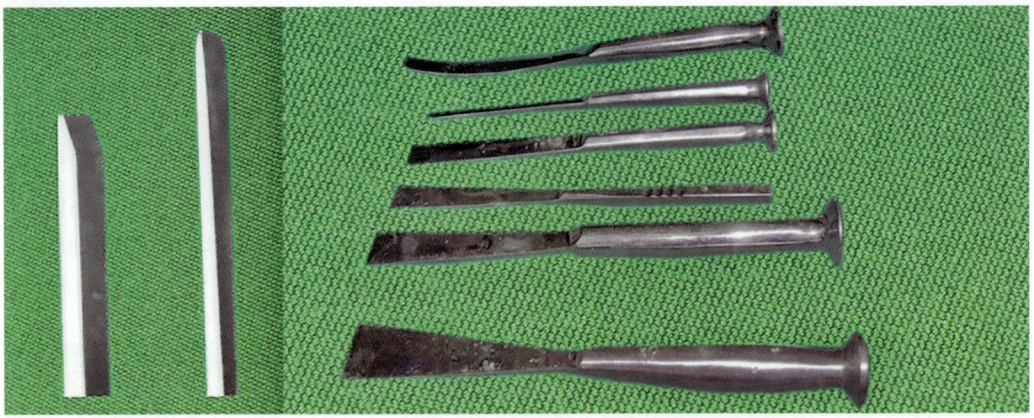

Osteotome

BONE CUTTER
Indications

- To cut sharp bony margins following extractions or surgical procedures.
- To cut sharp ridge projections during alveoloplasty procedures.

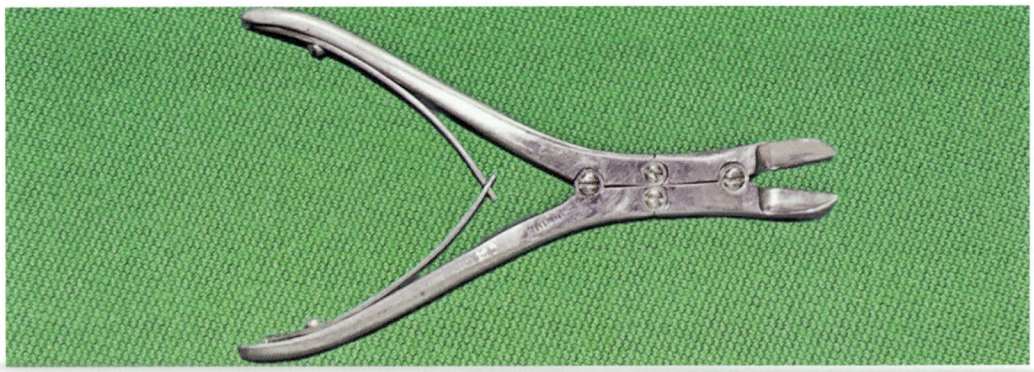

Bone cutter

DOYEN'S RIB SHEAR
Indication

- Used for rib cutting during rib harvesting procedure.

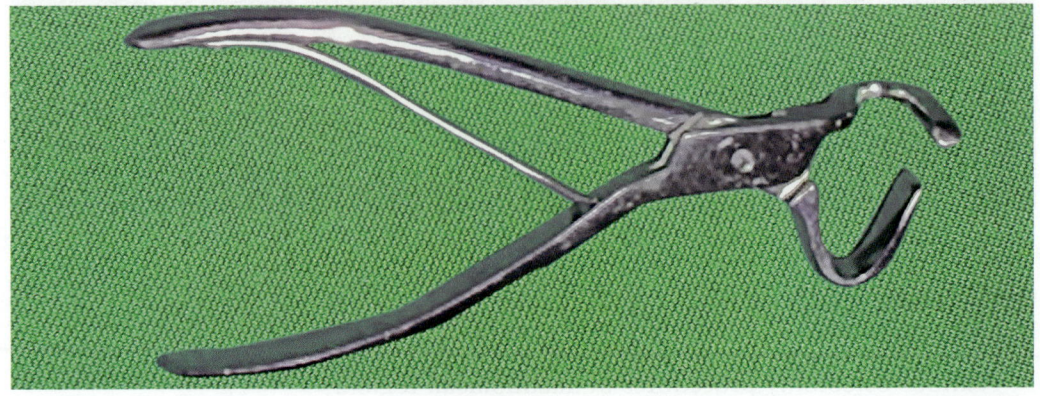

Doyen's rib shear

BONE GOUGE

Indications

- To make a window in anterior border of maxillary sinus (in Caldwell Luc surgery).
- To remove cancellous bone graft material/irregular pieces of bone.

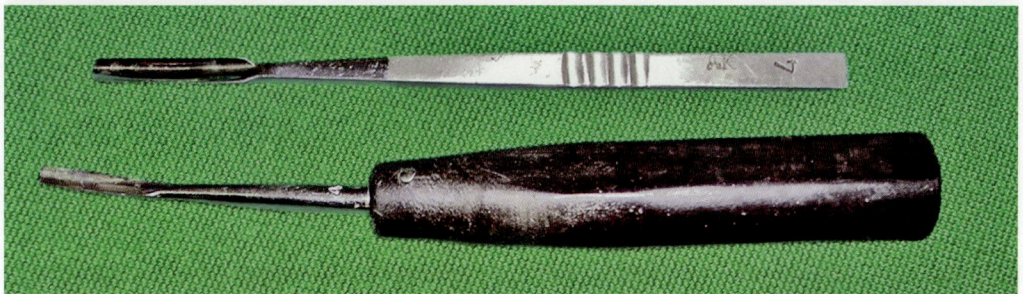

Bone gouge

INSTRUMENTS FOR INTERMAXILLARY FIXATION

WIRE TWISTER

Indication

- This instrument is used for holding wire, passing it interdentally or through bone for dentoalveolar wiring or transosseous wiring.

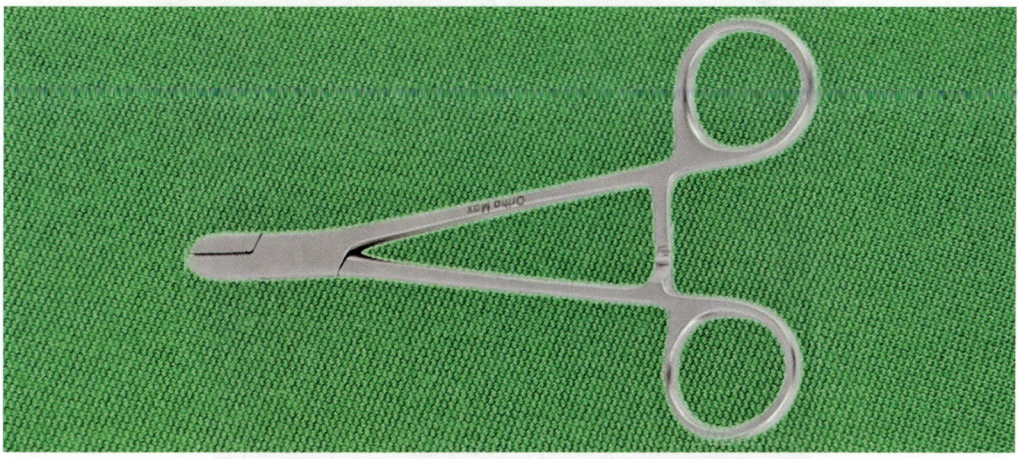

Wire twister

WIRE CUTTER

Indication

- A heavy wire cutter is used for cutting the ends of the twisted or stretched wire.

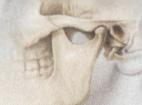

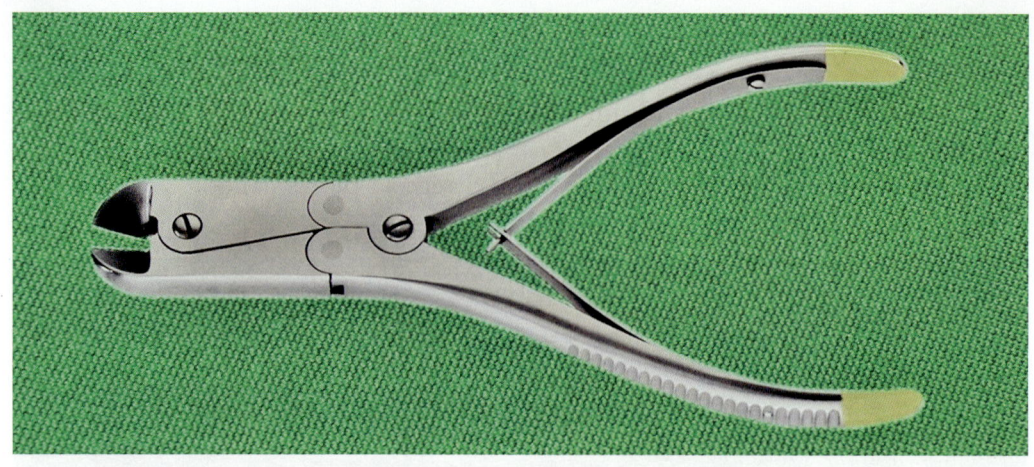

Wire cutter

INSTRUMENTS FOR INTERNAL FIXATION

TITANIUM SCREWS

It has a conical screw head that facilitates alignment of the locking screw in the threaded plate hole to provide a secure screw/plate construct. Cross slot at the top for

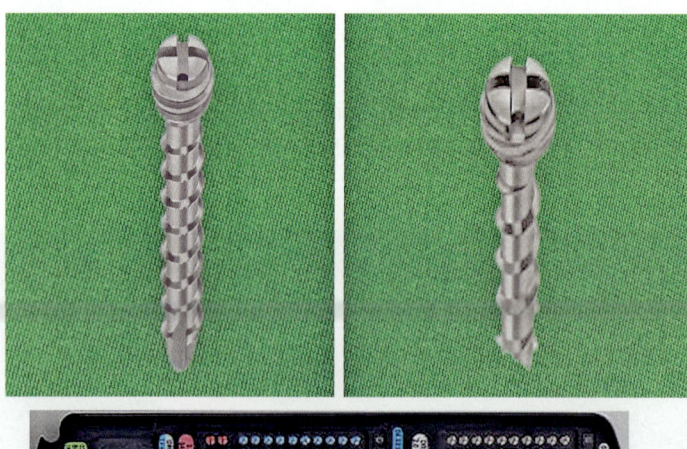

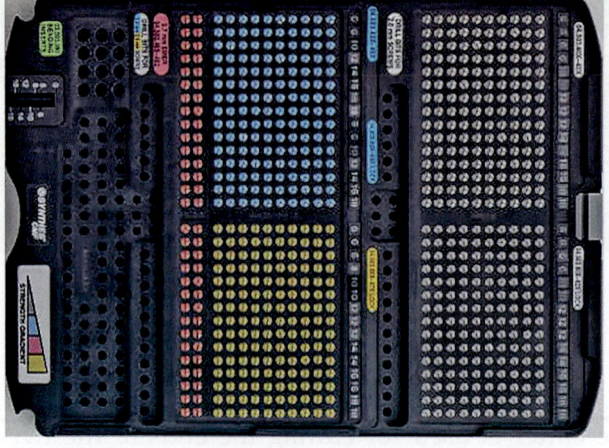

Titanium screws

screw engagement and retention. Available in different diameters and lengths, e.g. 1 mm, 1.5 mm, 2 mm, 2.5 mm diameter and 4 mm, 6 mm, and 8 mm in length. All screws have 1.0 mm pitch for fast insertion. Variety of designs are available, e.g. locking screw, non-locking screw. Made from titanium alloy (Ti-6Al-7Nb). A screw has a core about which is wrapped a spiral surface.

Indication

- It is used to stabilize the plates and anatomic reduction of fracture site.

TITANIUM PLATES (MONOCORTICAL)

It is available in a variety of sizes. The dimensions can be 1 mm, 1.5 mm, 2 mm, 2.5 mm, 2.8 mm in thickness, etc. Made from pure titanium. Rounded plate profiles and edges. Conical locking holes allow greater off-axis insertion tolerance and better thread engagement. All plates having feature of countersink for easy locating of cannula. It is available in various forms like straight, curved, L-shaped according to the need. Available as locking plates and non-locking plates. Plates in the form of mesh to reconstruct the floor of orbit. 3D plates are also available for anatomic reduction. Titanium plates are used to hold the fracture segments in anatomic position. 1 mm,

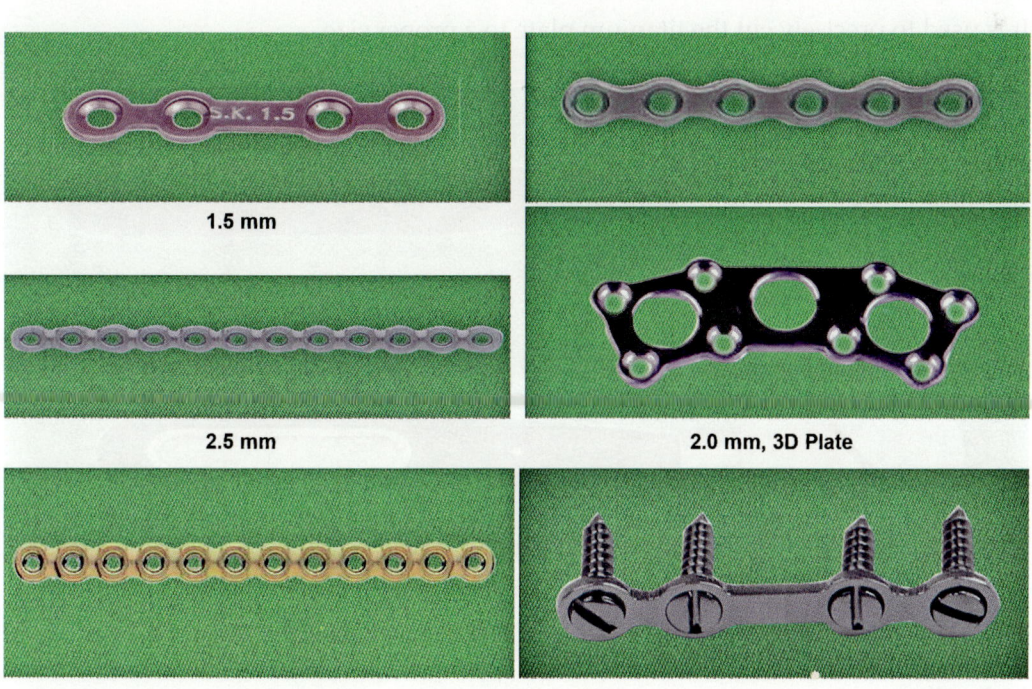

1.5 mm

2.5 mm

2.0 mm, 3D Plate

2.8 mm locking plates

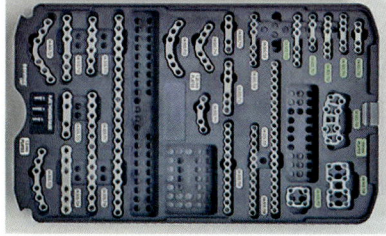
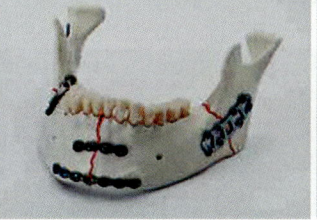
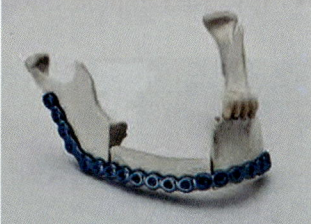

Titanium plates (monocortical)

1.5 mm, 2 mm, titanium plates are used maxillofacial trauma and 2.5 mm, 2.8 mm thickness plates are used for primary mandibular reconstruction with bone grafts.

SCREW DRIVER

Indication

- It is used to tighten the titanium screw during fracture fixation

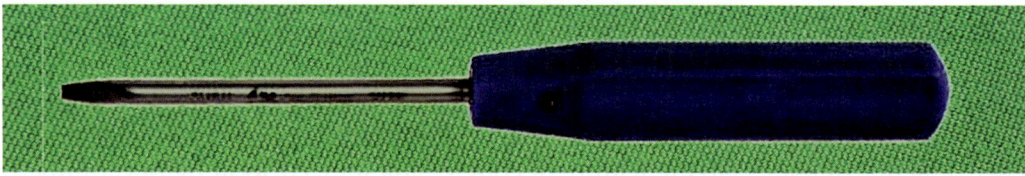

Screw driver

PLATE CUTTERS IN PAIRS

Indication

It is used to precisely cut the titanium plate to a proper size.

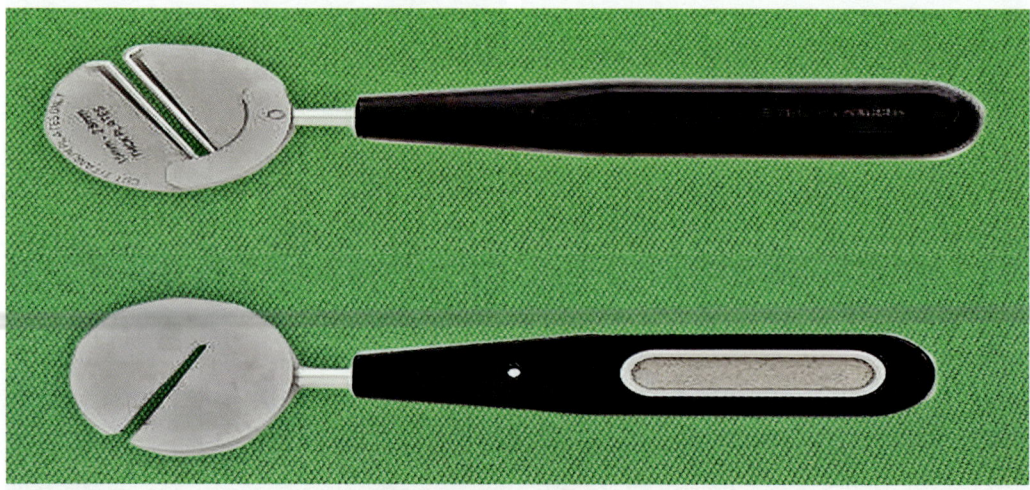

Plate cutters in pairs

SELF-RETAINING SCREW DRIVER

Indication

- It is used to hold the screw.

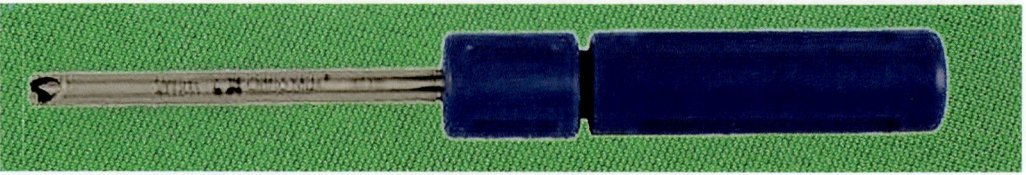

Self-retaining screw driver

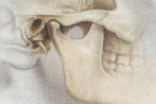
PLATE BENDING PLIERS
Indication
- It is used to bend titanium plate according to the anatomy of bone during fracture reduction.

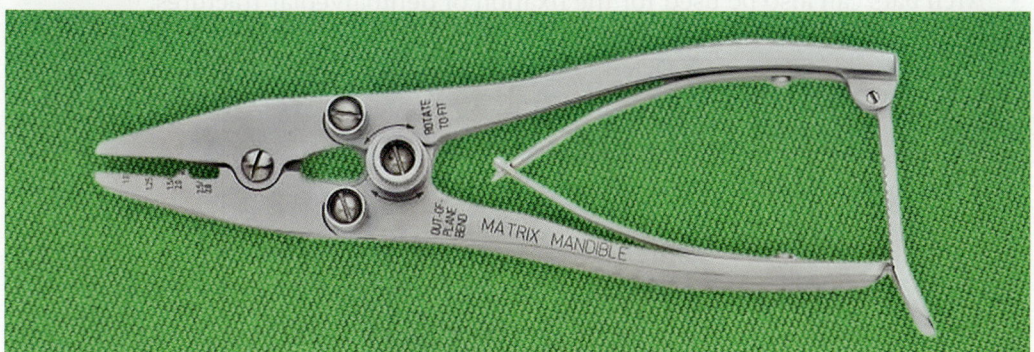

Plate bending pliers

MINI PLATE HOLDER
Indication
- It is used to hold the mini plates.

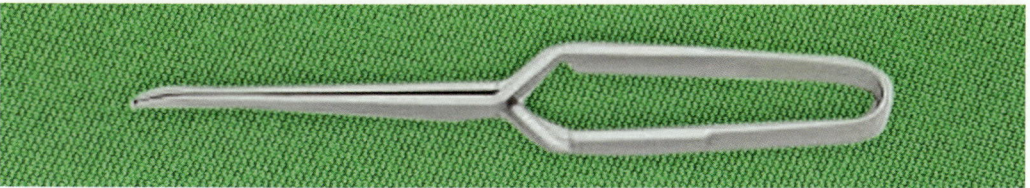

Mini plate holder

PLATE INTRODUCING FORCEPS
Indication
- It is used to introduce the plate at fracture site during surgery.

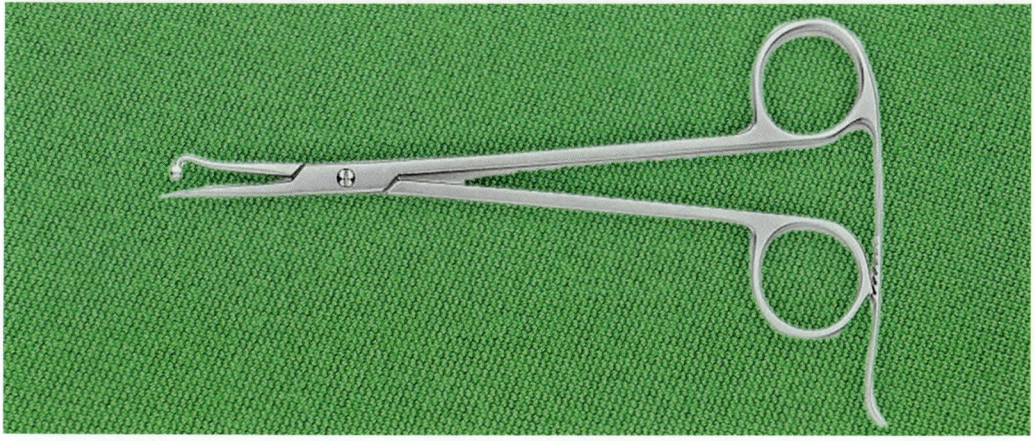

Plate introducing forceps

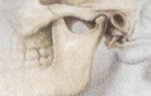

ERICH'S ARCH BAR

Indications

- Upper and lower arch bars may be placed and wired together keeping the teeth in occlusion for maxillomandibular fixation.
- Arch bars can also be used for the fixation of dentoalveolar fractures.

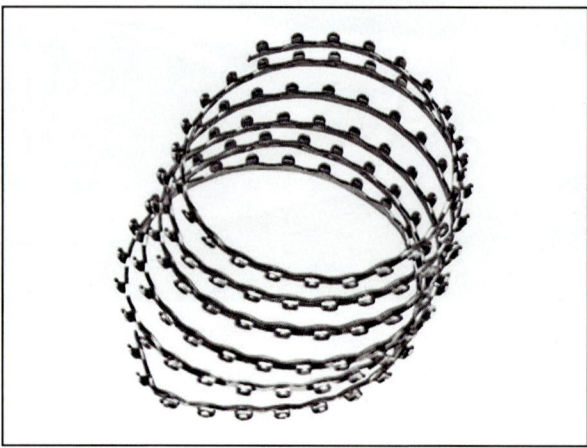

Erich's arch bar

TRANSBUCCAL TROCAR SYSTEM

Identifying Features

- The handle of trocar is broad and sturdy with indentation for proper grip.
- It has C-shaped malleable cheek retractor which is adapted to the cheek and corner of mouth.

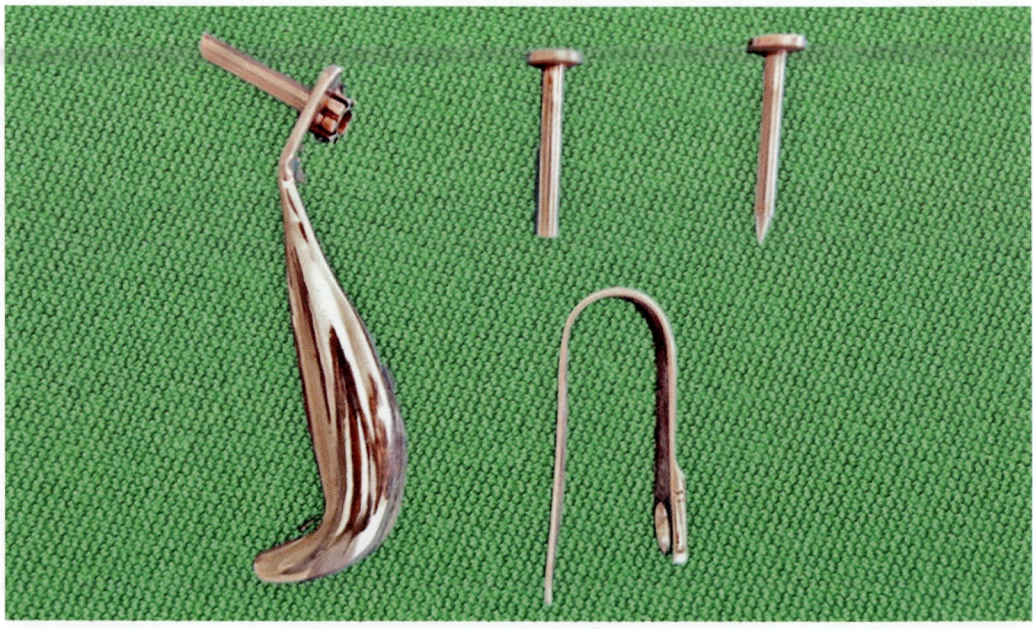

Transbuccal trocar system

- It has two collars, one is present intraorally and the other is extraorally.
- Both collars get adapted to the working end of trocar on the other side.
- A drill guide is having long, cylinder, and hollow working end, through which the drill bit is passed to prepare a hole on either side of fracture line.
- The other end of drill guide has a flat disk-shaped structure which supports the working end. It guides the drill bit to reach the fracture line.
- Trocar cannula has long, cylindrical pointed working end to explore the soft tissue before application of trocar drill.

Indication

- It is used for transbuccal approach in the management of mandibular angle and ramus fracture.

INSTRUMENTS FOR CLOSURE

NEEDLE HOLDER

Adson tissue forceps

Dean's suture cutting scissor

Note: Detailed description in chapter on General Surgical Instruments.

Orthognathic Instruments

Jeevan Khatri, Murali Mohan, M Ehtaihsham

OSTEOTOME
Identifying Features

- Similar to chisel but the edges of working tip is bi-beveled.
- It splits bone rather than cutting or chipping it.

Indications

- Osteotomy procedures in orthognathic surgeries.
- Removal/recontouring of bone.

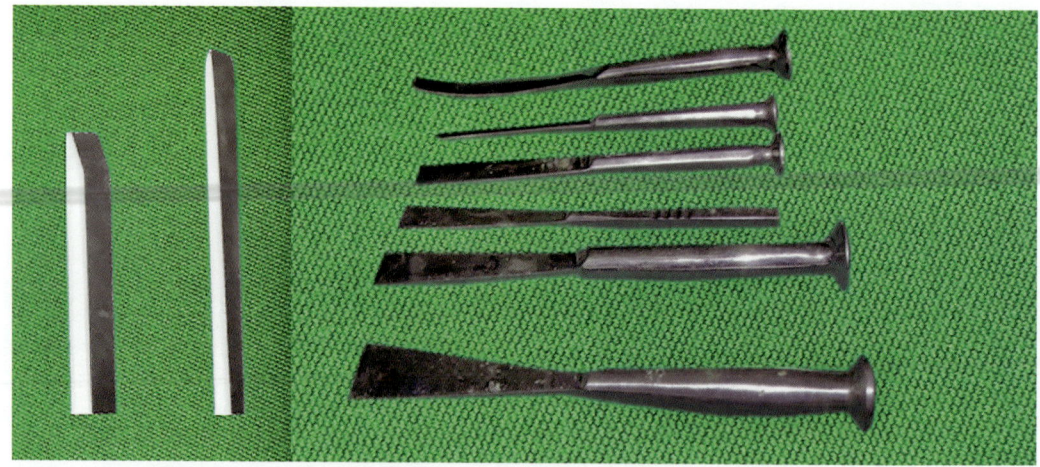

Osteotome

PTERYGOID OSTEOTOME
Identifying Features

- It has long, flat and curved working blade.
- Handle is broad and circular in design.

Practise Note

- Proper orientation is assured by placing an index finger on palate at hamular notch to palpate the osteotome tip prior to malleting.

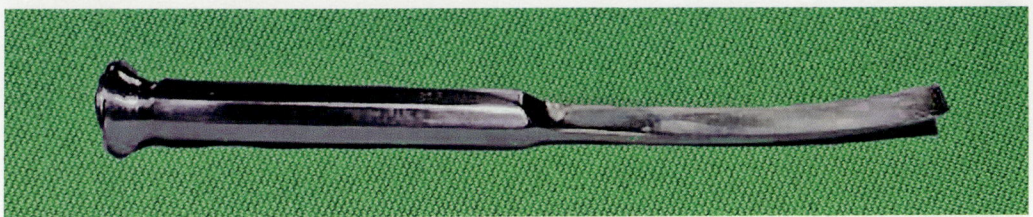

Pterygoid osteotome

Indication

- In Lefort–I osteotomies separation of maxilla from pterygoid plates is done with pterygoid osteotome directed medially and anteriorly at the lowest part of the junction of maxilla and pterygoid plate.

TEISSER'S MAXILLA MOBILISER

Indication

- Used to separate bony fragments after completion of the osteotomy cuts.

To check separation of fragments from pterygoid plates during downward fracture of maxilla in Le Fort-I osteotomies.

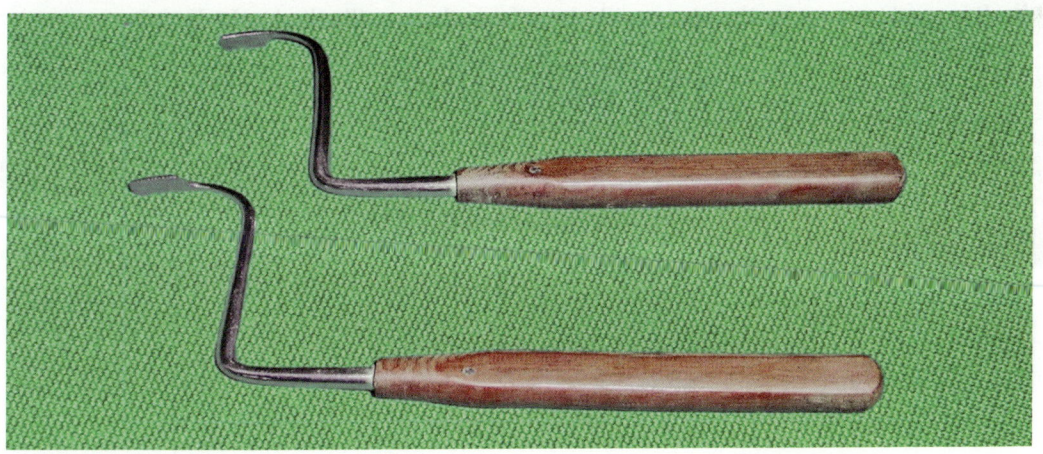

Teisser's maxilla mobiliser

SMITH SPREADER

Identifying Features

- It has 3 blades at working end.
- The handle is with double spring, activated by spring mechanism. The blades are separated when the handles are squeezed.
- Also available in curved design that has more advantages than straight one.

Indications

- Used to separate bony fragments after completion of the osteotomy cut.
- To check separation of fragments during downward fracture of maxilla/sagittal split osteotomy procedure.

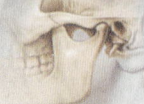

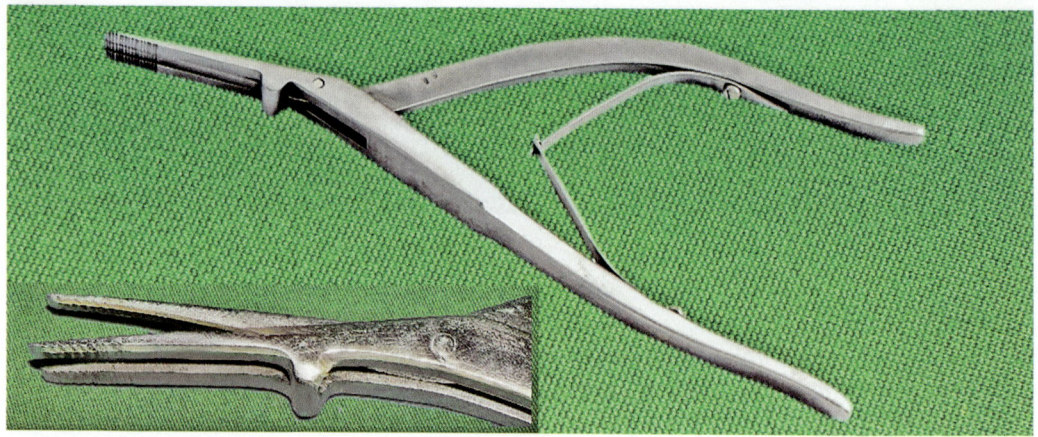

Smith spreader

PTERYGOID CHISEL

Identifying features

- It is a flat instrument having bevel on one side of the working end.

Indication

- It is used to separate the pterygoid plates from the maxilla during Le Fort-I osteotomy procedure.

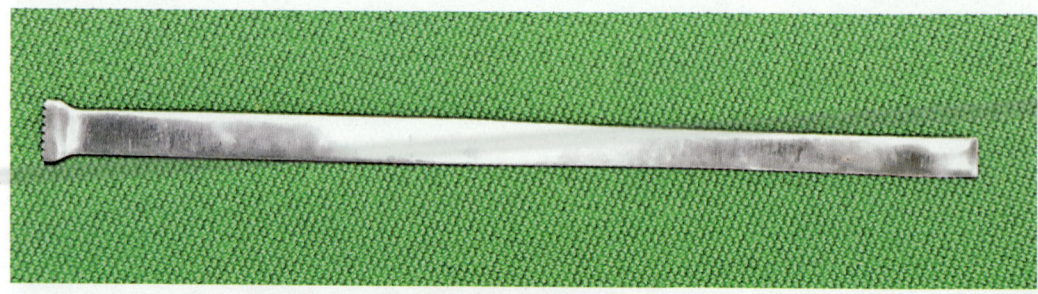

Pterygoid chisel

OSCILLATING SAW AND HANDPIECE

Identifying Features

Unit consists of
- Regulator, foot control and cable.
- Handpiece
  - Electric powered
  - Pneumatic powered (uses compressed air at 90–110 psi pressure) saw with hand pieces speed of 10,000–1 lac rpm can be achieved.

Different kinds of saws available for various types of osteotomy.

Sagittal saw moves side to side (5–6° arc), used for wedge/transverse osteotomy. Oscillating saw oscillates (5–6° arc), used for curved/straight osteotomy. Reciprocating saw moves to and fro (2.4 mm), used for short/long osteotomy.

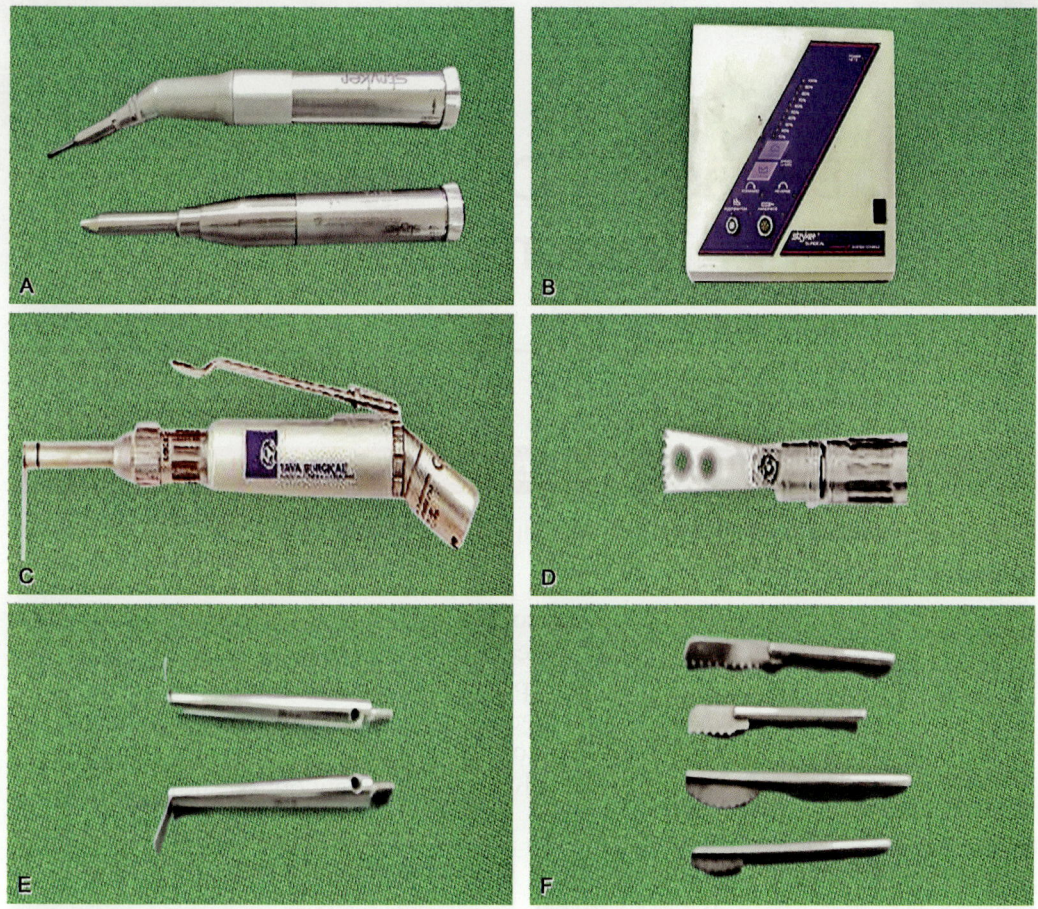

Oscillating saw and handpiece

Indication

It gives ease of cutting bone with precision because of different shape/movements of saw, used during osteotomy procedure in orthognathic surgeries like Le Fort I, II, and BSSO.

Distraction Osteogenesis Instruments

SC Bhoyar, Shoeb Jendi

EXTRAORAL DISTRACTORS

EXTERNAL MANDIBULAR DISTRACTOR—UNIDIRECTIONAL

Identifying Features

- The unidirectional mandibular distractor has two clamps—a rotating clamp and a sliding clamp, both connected to the geared distractor.
- Each clamp contains a pair of fixation pins for attachment.
- Similar to the Hoffman Mini Lengthener, rotation and sliding of clamps allows the apparatus to adapt the shape and size of mandible.
- Distraction is performed by turning advancement screw on the sliding clamp.

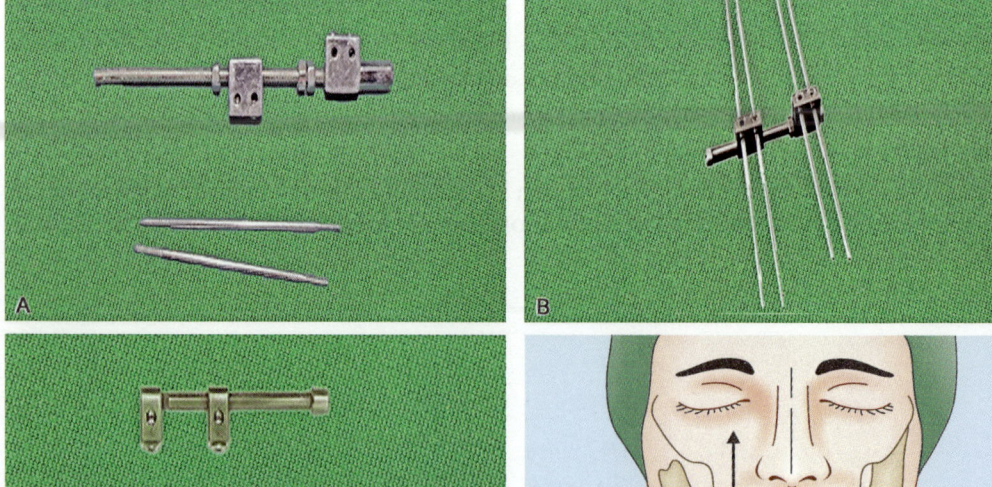

External mandibular distractor—unidirectional

Indication

- It is used for complete correction of linear discrepancies only.

EXTERNAL MANDIBULAR DISTRACTOR—BIDIRECTIONAL
Identifying Features

- The bidirectional distractor has two distractor rods.
- It has three clamps with each clamp containing a pair of fixation pins for attachment.
- Both distractor rods are connected to the sliding circular metal device.

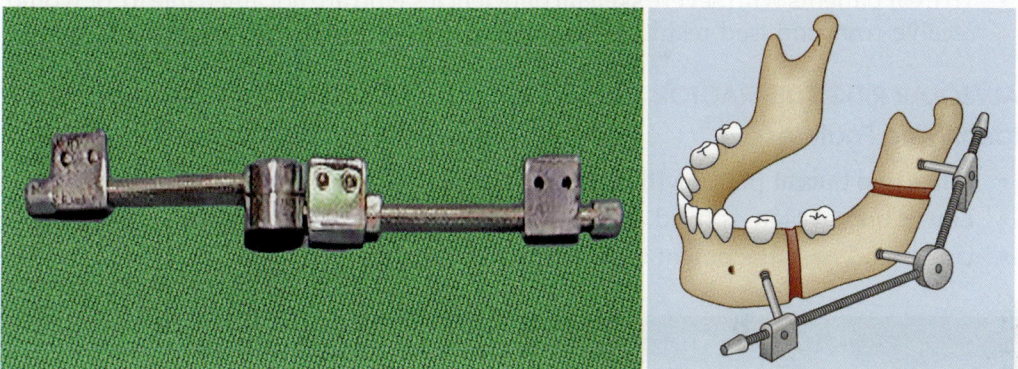

External mandibular distractor—bidirectional

Indication

It is used for complete correction of vertical and horizontal deficiencies of mandible simultaneously.

EXTERNAL MIDFACE DISTRACTOR
Identifying Features

- It has a metal framework with distraction segment at the top.
- It has carbon rods, 120 mm in length, horizontally placed to connect right and left framework.

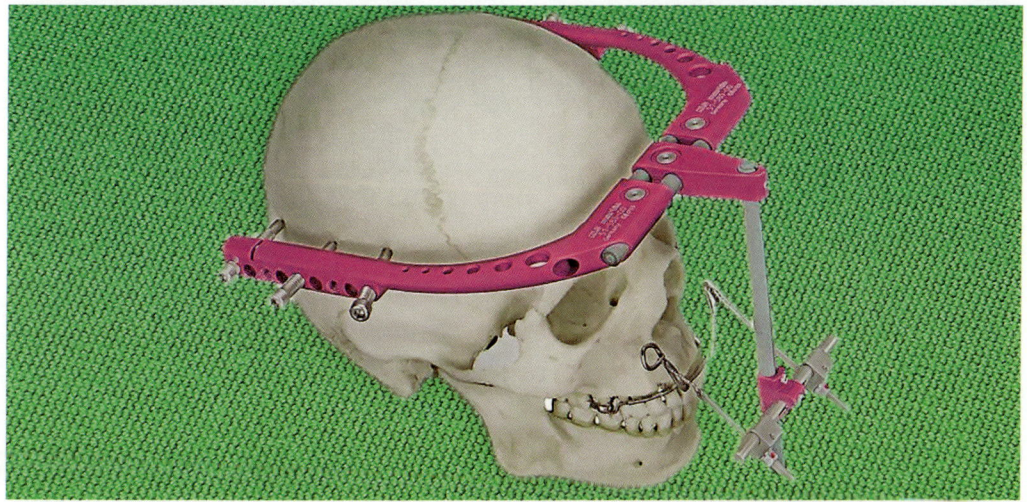

External midface distractor

- It has another vertical carbon rod of 150 mm in length.
- The connection to the occlusal level can be achieved by an intraoral splint.
- Vertical carbon rod support the horizontal assembly including horizontal cross bar, holder, 2 spindle units and fixation screws (45 mm to cranial bones).

Indications

- It is used to gradually lengthen the midface at the Le Fort I, II, and III levels (including monobloc).
- To treat patients with severe skeletal deficiencies who are not amenable to, or would receive compromised results with conventional orthognathic surgery.

ALVEOLAR RIDGE DISTRACTOR

Identifying Features

- It has two buccal plates with a central distraction rod.
- Lower buccal plate is fixed and the upper buccal plate is movable.
- Upper end has attachment to fit the internal surface of activator.

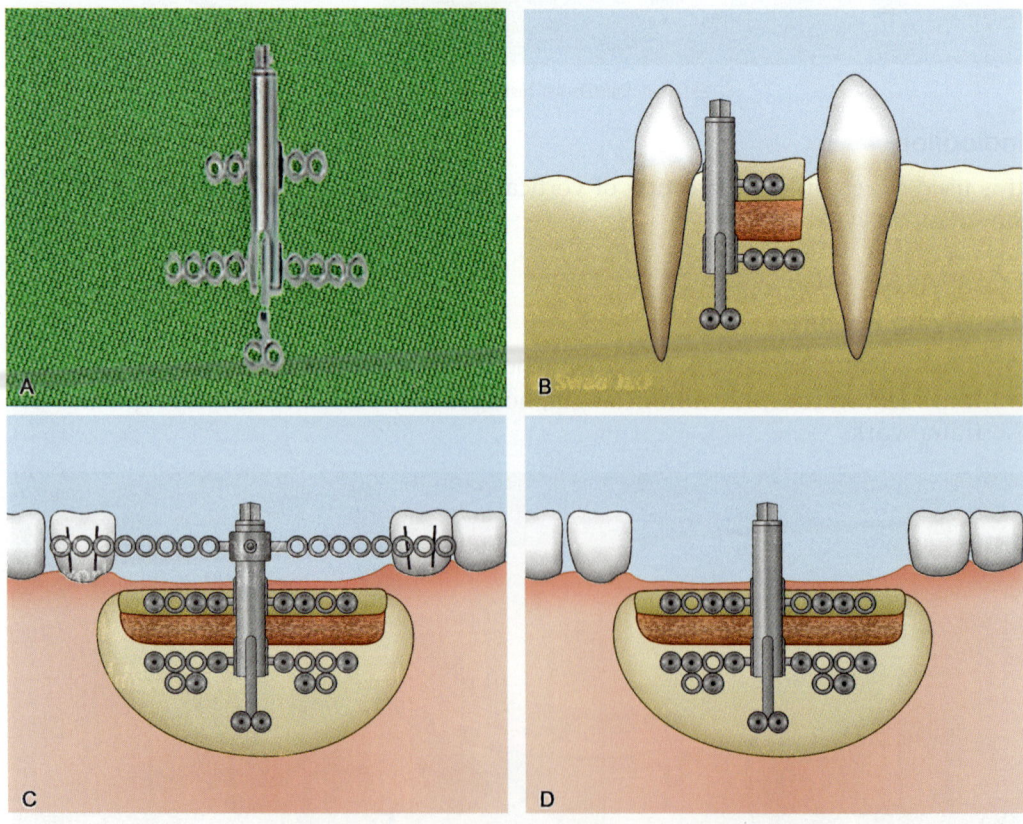

Alveolar ridge distractor

Indications

- It is used for the augmentation of the maxillary and mandibular alveolar ridge.
- Local vertical ridge defect and ankylosed teeth.

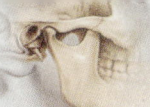

INTRA-ORAL RAMUS DISTRACTOR
Identifying Features
- Fixed block, with three holes bone plates.
- Movable block, with three holes bone plates.
- Threaded central rod, with extension for activation.
- Two guided supporting rods and stabilizing plate holding the threads.

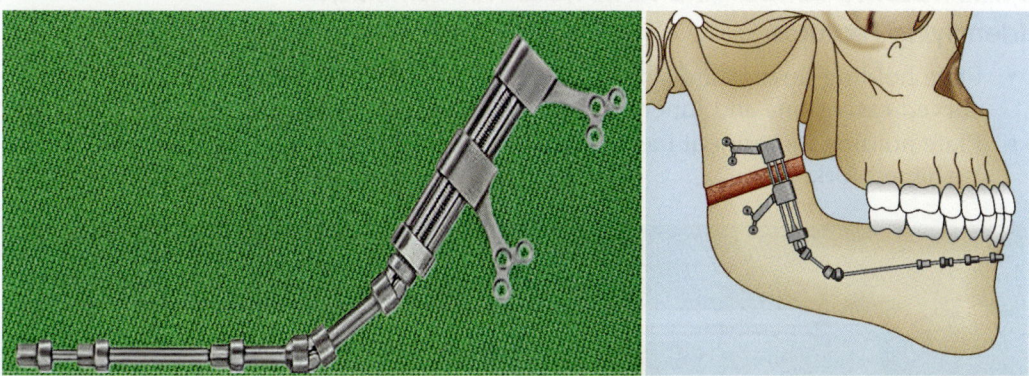

Intra-oral ramus distractor

Indication
- This distractor is used to treat vertical deficiencies of mandible.

MAXILLARY DISTRACTION DEVICE
Identifying Features
- Upper bone plate—hexagonal in shape and easily adaptable, it is adapted to the malar bone/buttress and fixed to the zygomatic buttress of maxilla above the osteotomy cut and is fixed with stainless steel screws (8–10 mm in length of 2 mm diameter).
- Lower bone plate—straight and also easily adaptable, it is fixed to the alveolar process of maxilla 2 to 3 mm above the root apices of teeth below the osteotomy cut with stainless steel screws (8 to 10 mm in length, 2 mm in diameter).

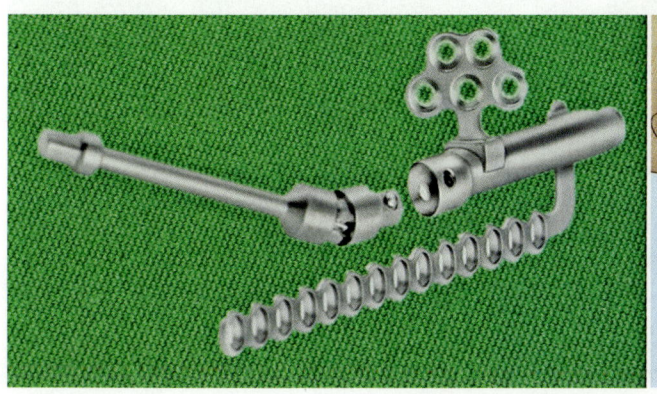
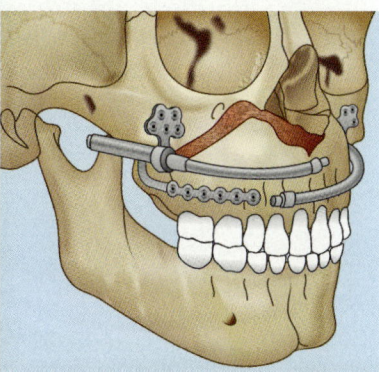

Maxillary distraction device

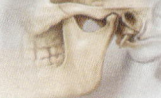

- Activation port—consists of the activation screw present intra-orally. It is to be activated daily 1 mm/day as per the requirement of the case.
- Activation of device.

Indication

- It is used for full correction of midface deficiency.

PLATE HOLDING FORCEP AND PLATE HOLDING INSTRUMENT
Identifying Features

- Plate holding forceps are similar to cotton forceps with working end having two curved extensions and inner surface serrations.
- Plate holding instrument has one working end with rounded tip and another has V-shaped fork.

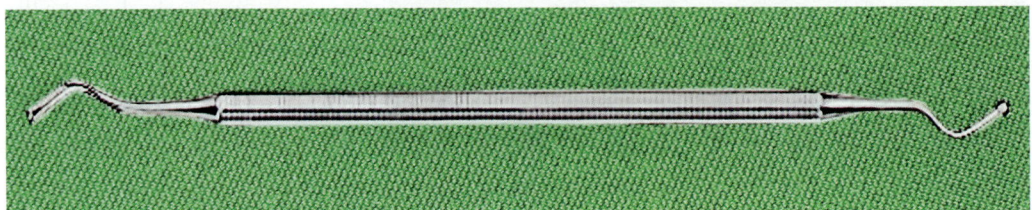

Plate holding forceps and plate holding instrument

Indication

- To hold the plate during operative procedure.

MODELING PLIERS
Identifying Features

- It is heavy instrument with working ends having pointed tips.
- The working blades have serrations.

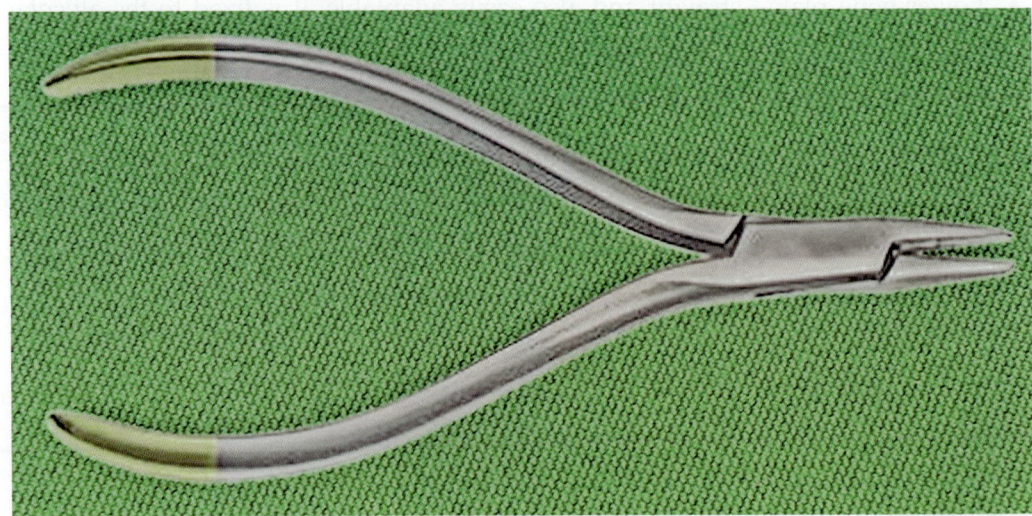

Modeling pliers

Indication

- To mould the plates according to the anatomy.

ACTIVATOR MEASURING DEVICE
Identifying Features

- It is measuring device with marking that ranges from 10 to 70 mm.

Indication

- It is used to measure amount of distraction in millimeters.

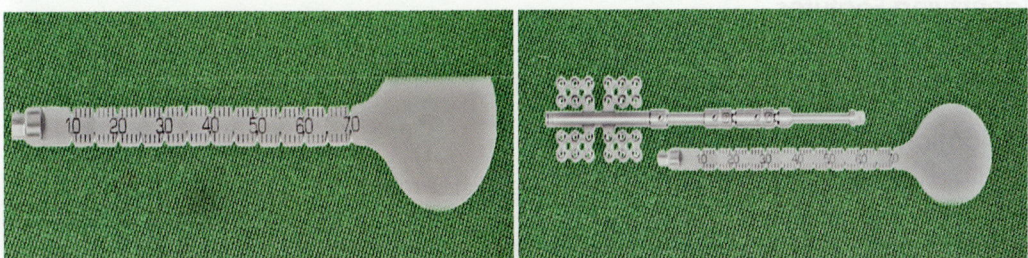

Activator measuring device

ACTIVATION ARM DISCONNECTION FORCEPS
Identifying Features

- It is forcep type with working end having 2 round projections on inner surface of the tip.

Indication

- It is used to disconnect the activation arm.

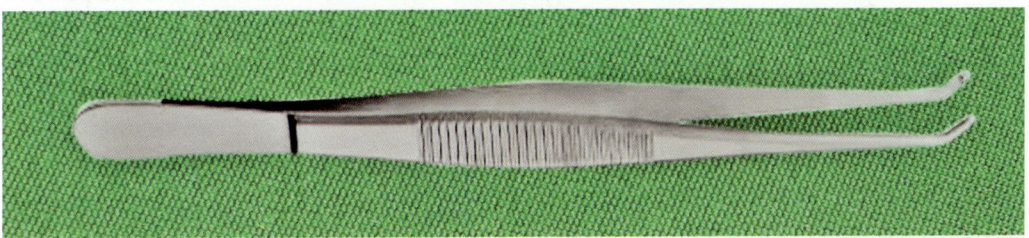

Activation arm disconnection forceps

SCREW DRIVER FOR EXTERNAL HEXAGONAL DISTRACTOR TYPE
Identifying Features

- The working end is hexagonal in type.
- Handle of instrument is round with central indentations.

Indication

- It is used to apply to the screw during external distractor placement.

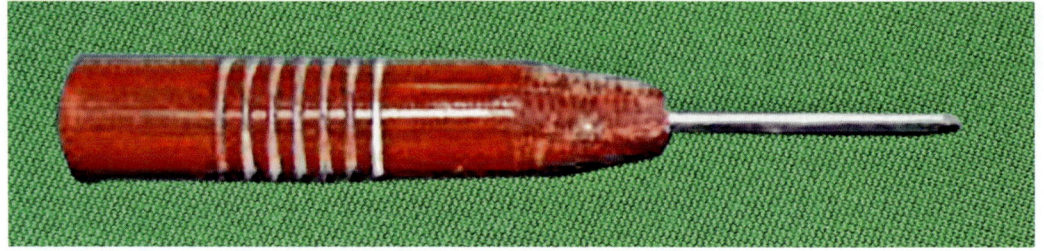

Screw driver for external hexagonal distractor type

SCHANZ SCREWS

Identifying Features

- Schanz screws with working ends having pointed tip.
- Body is cylindrical and tip has serrations.

Indication

- It is used to stabilize the distractor used extraorally.

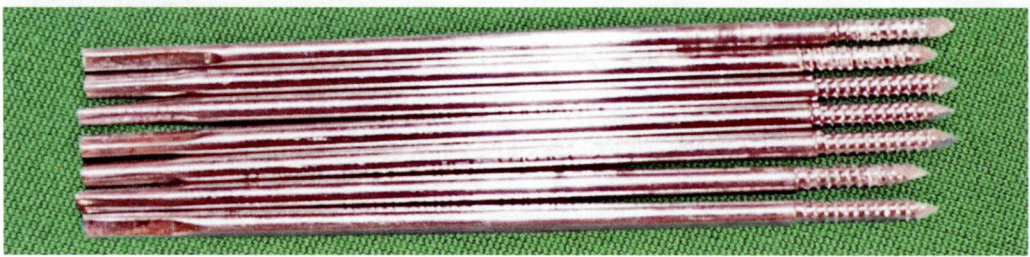

Schanz screws

PLATE CUTTER

Identifying Features

- It is heavy instrument with working end having slot to accommodate the plate.
- Handle has leaf spring.

Indication

- It is used to cut the plates during placement.

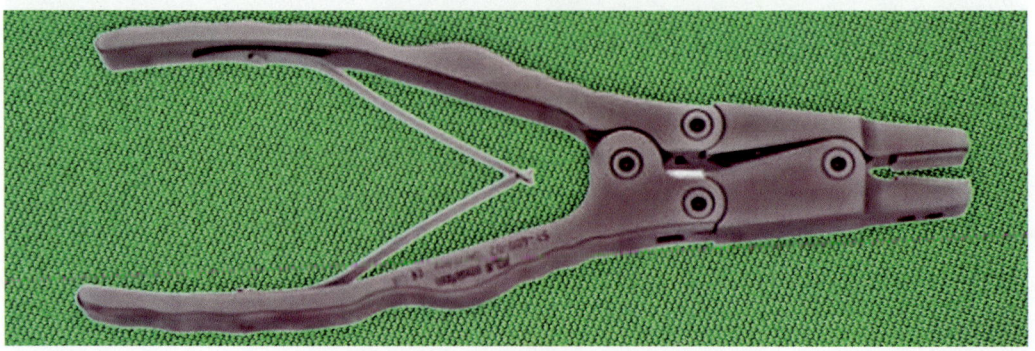

Plate cutter

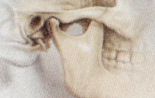
MICRO IMPLANT (SCREWS)
Identifying Features
- Monocortical micro-implant with serration at whole body.
- Inner end of micro-implant has pointed tip and outer end has slot for screw driver.

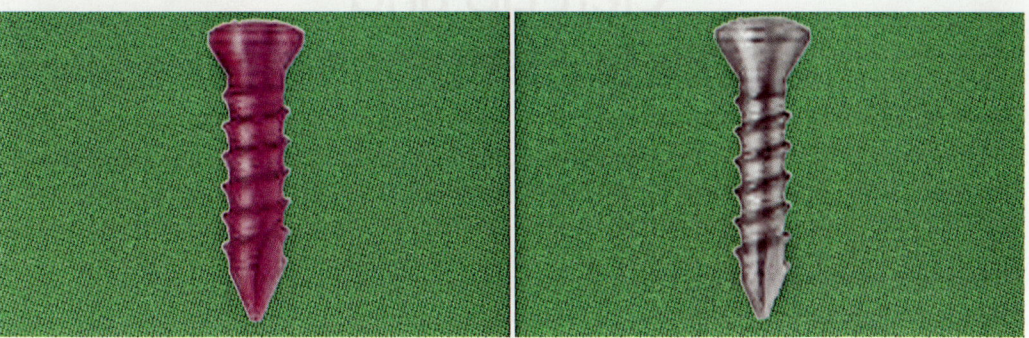

Micro implant (screws)

Indication
- It is used to stabilize the distractor used intraorally.

Cleft Lip and Palate Instruments

Mohammad Yaseen, Vithal Lahane, Priyanka Samel

DINGMAN MOUTH GAG WITH BLADES

Identifying Features

- It is a closed rectangular metallic frame having attachments on the caudal side on which an adjustable tongue retractor is mounted in the centre which supports the gag inferiorly and holds an endotracheal tube over the tongue.

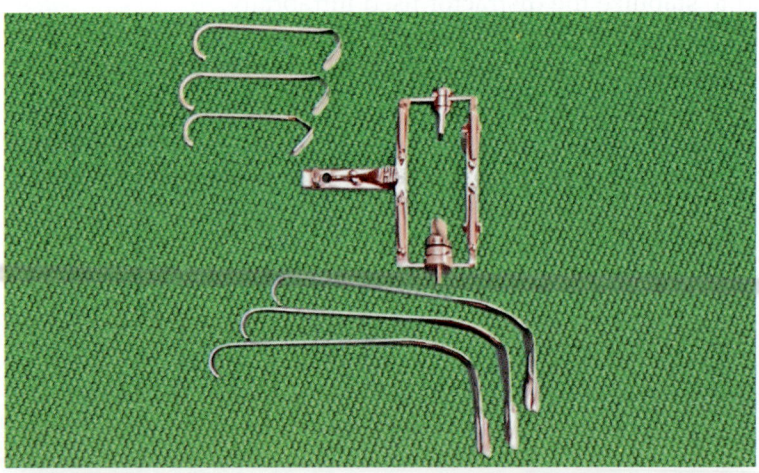

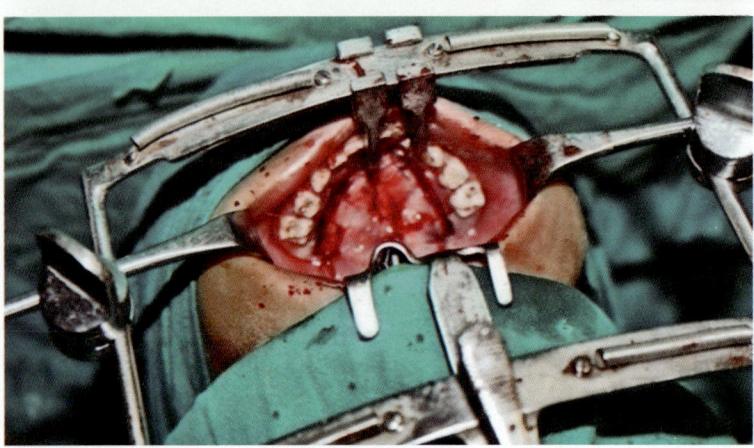

Dingman mouth gag with blades

- It has two clamps on either side of the cephalad side for adjusting the pair of alveolar bar that rests on the alveolar ridge.
- These alveolar bars co-act with tongue retractor to retain jaw in desired position.
- The alveolar bars can be adjusted both for axial rotation and longitudinal sliding.

Indications

- To keep the mouth open during cleft lip and palate surgery under general anaesthesia.
- To keep mouth open during prolonged intraoral surgeries under local anesthesia.

CLEFT PALATE RASPATORY

Identifying Features

- The working end of raspatory is broad and flat.
- It may be straight or curved at the tip.
- It may be single or double ended.

Different Patterns of Raspatory

- Cleft raspatory Barsky type.
- Cleft raspatory French type.

Indication

- It is used to elevate the palatal mucoperiosteum, while mobilizing the flaps for cleft palate repair.

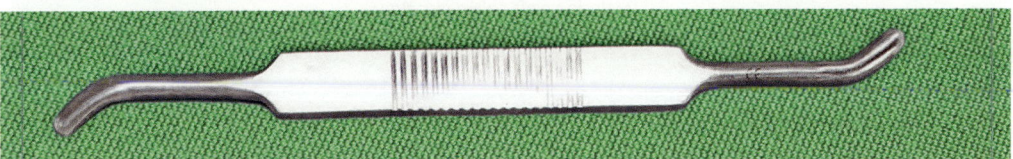

(a) Barsky type of raspatory (double ended)

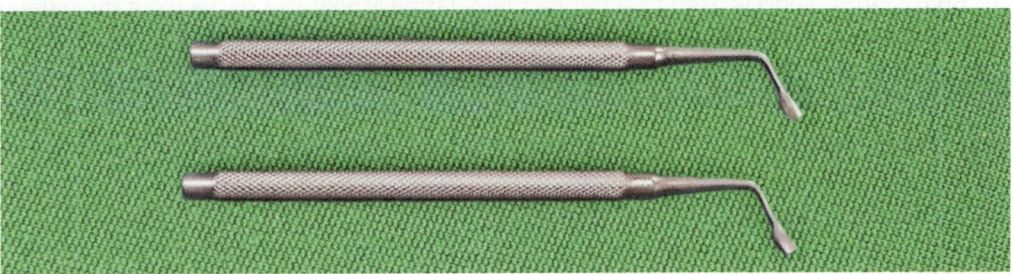

(b) French type of raspatory

CLEFT PALATE RASPATORY—CURVED UP AND DOWN

Identifying Features

- It has a long working blade with tips curved up and down.
- It has a flat handle.

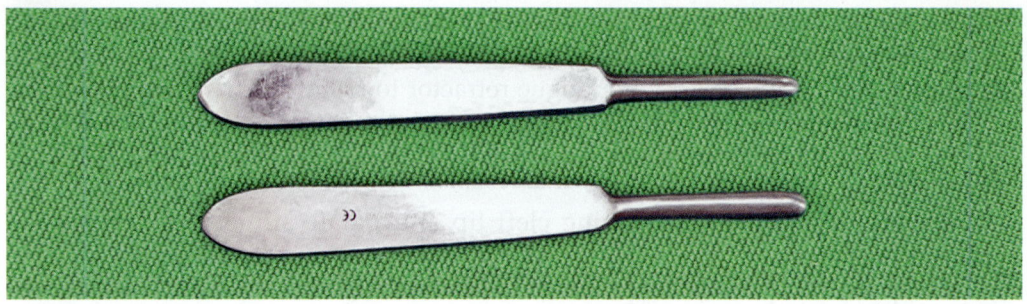

Cleft palate raspatory (curved pattern)

Indication

- It is used in cleft palate surgery to elevate the palatal mucoperiosteum from the palate.

MCINDOE CLEFT PALATE RASPATORY
Identifying Features

- It has two working ends—one is curved sharp pointed blade and the other one has broad flat offset blade.

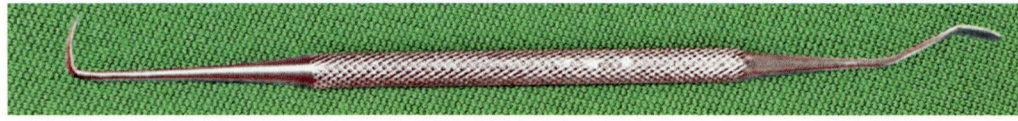

McIndoe cleft palate raspatory

Parts

- Blade, shank and handle
- The handle is round with the shank tapering towards blade.

Indication

- Sharp curved end is used to separate the palatine artery and nerve from the palatal soft tissue and the other end to elevate mucoperiosteal flap from palate.

BARSKY PHARYNGEAL FLAP ELEVATOR
Identifying Features

- It has double ended angled blade.
- It has round handle.
- The blades are 3 mm and 5 mm long.

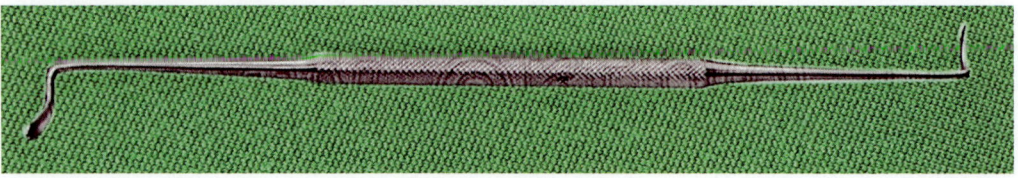

Barsky pharyngeal flap elevator

Indication

- It is used for the elevation of pharyngeal flap during cleft lip and palate surgery in patients with velopharyngeal incompetence.

CLEFT PALATE KNIFE—TRIANGULAR

Identifying Features

- It has sharp pointed blade which is at right angle to shank.
- Handle is round with tapered smooth shank.

Indication

- It is used to incise the palatal mucosa in the cleft palate surgery.

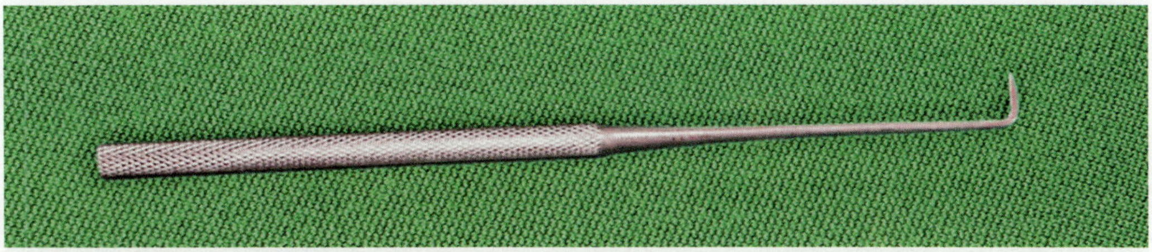

Cleft palate knife (triangular pattern)

CRONIN CLEFT PALATE ELEVATOR

Identifying Features

- It has angulated flat blade that allows for delicate handling of the soft tissues.
- It is available in different sizes based on the type of surgical field.

Indications

- It is commonly used tool in cleft palate reconstructive surgery.
- It is used to lift the mucoperiosteal flap once the incision is made along the oral and the nasal mucosa.

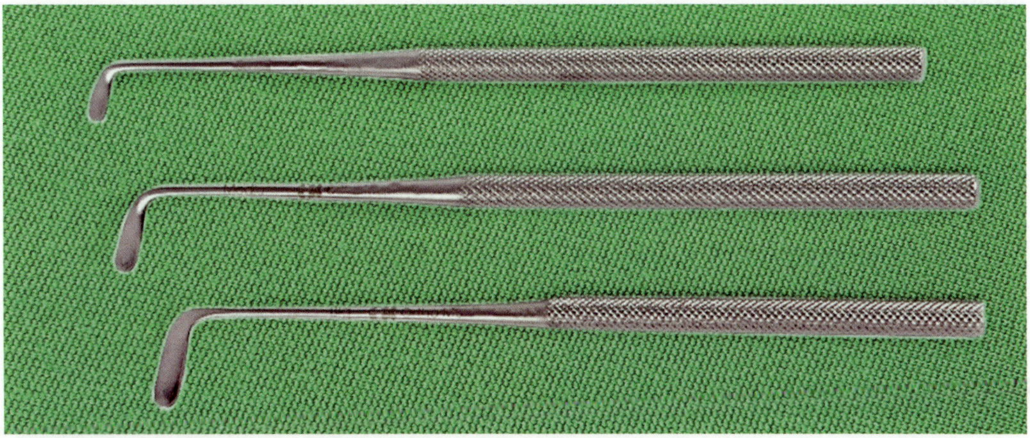

Cronin cleft palate elevator

MITCHELL TRIMMER

Identifying Features

• It is a double-ended instrument.

Parts

- Knife blade
- Spoon elevator
- Handle

Indication

- It is an ideal instrument for the trimming of palatal mucosa during cleft palate closure.

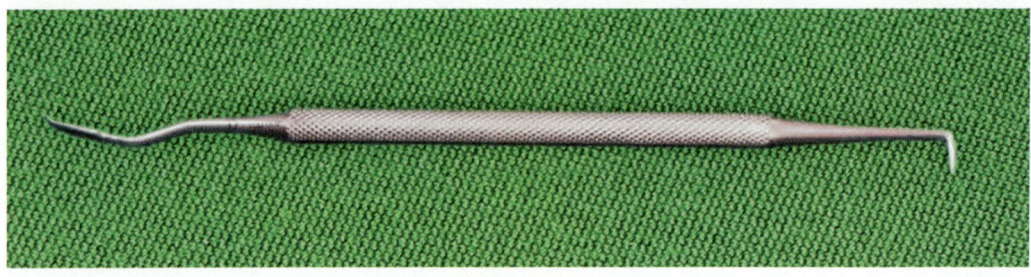

Mitchell trimmer

CLEFT PALATE HOOK

Identifying Features

- It is a single-ended instrument.

Parts

- Hook
- Shank
- Handle

Indication

- It is used for holding the mucosal and mucoperiosteal flap during cleft palate surgery.

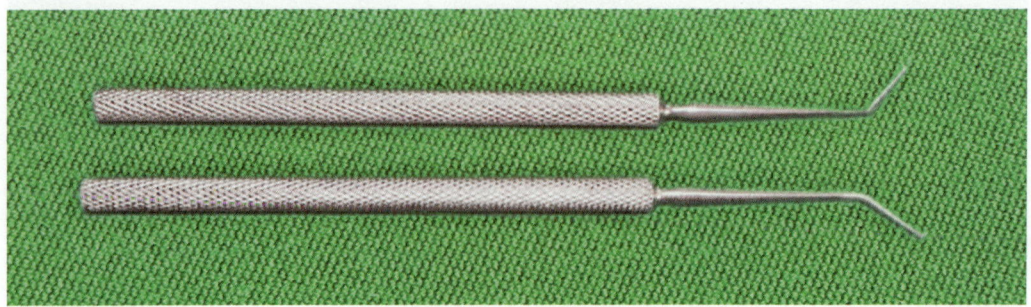

Cleft palate hook

PALATE DISSECTOR

Identifying Features

- It is a single-ended instrument.
- The blade is at an angle to the shank with round edge.

Parts

- Blade
- Shank
- Handle

Indication

- It is used in cleft palate surgery to elevate the mucoperiosteal flap.

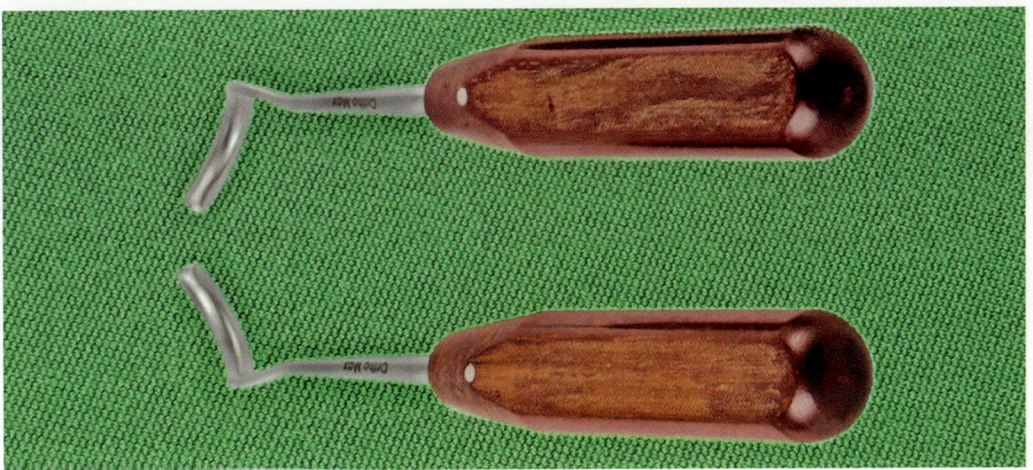

Palate dissector

MILLER'S BONE FILE

Identifying Features

- It is a double-ended instrument.
- The working end is flat with horizontal serrations.

Indication

- It is used for final smoothening of the hamulus process after fracturing in cleft palate surgery to preserve greater palatine neurovascular bundle.

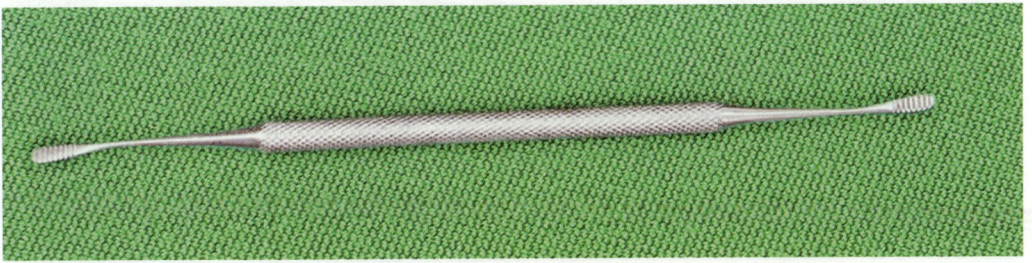

Miller's bone file

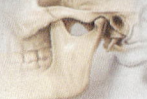

SPOON SHAPED ELEVATOR

Identifying Features

- It is a double-ended instrument.
- The blades are present at an angle to the shank.

Parts

- Blade
- Shank
- Handle

Indication

- It is used to elevate the right and left side palatal mucoperiosteal flaps during cleft palate surgery.

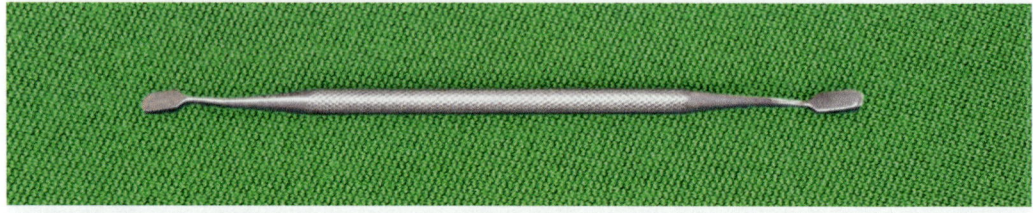

Spoon shaped elevator

CASTROVIEJO CALIPER

Identifying Features

- The handle has a screw for adjustment according to the scale.
- It has a sharp pointed working end.
- The other end has a measurement plate, with pointer that denotes the measurement in millimeters.

Indication

- It is used for marking the desired measurements before taking incision in cleft lip and palate surgery.

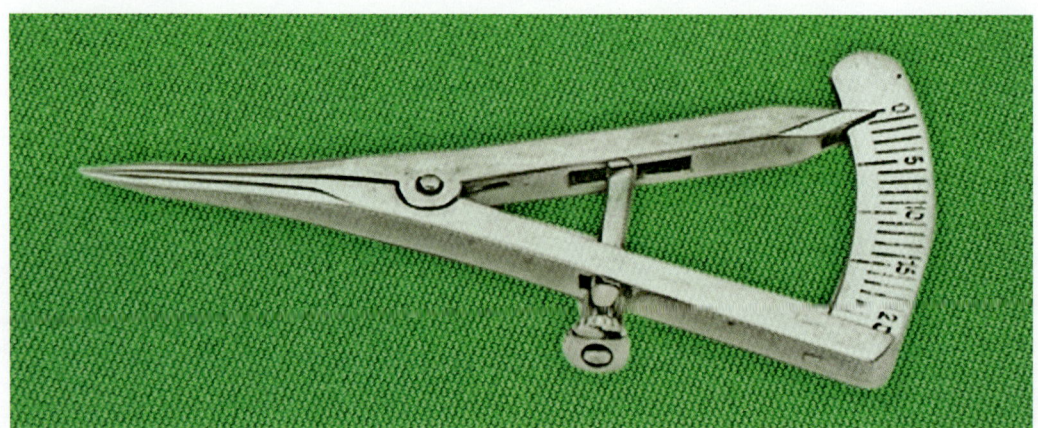

Castroviejo caliper

Rhinoplasty Instruments

Virendra Ghaisas, Sameer Shaikh

OSTEOTOMES

Identifying Features

- It is very fine straight, double-edged, with rounded corners and with recessed grip osteotome.
- The length of osteotome is 18 cm.
- It is available in different sizes like 2 mm, 3 mm, 4 mm, 6 mm of working blades.

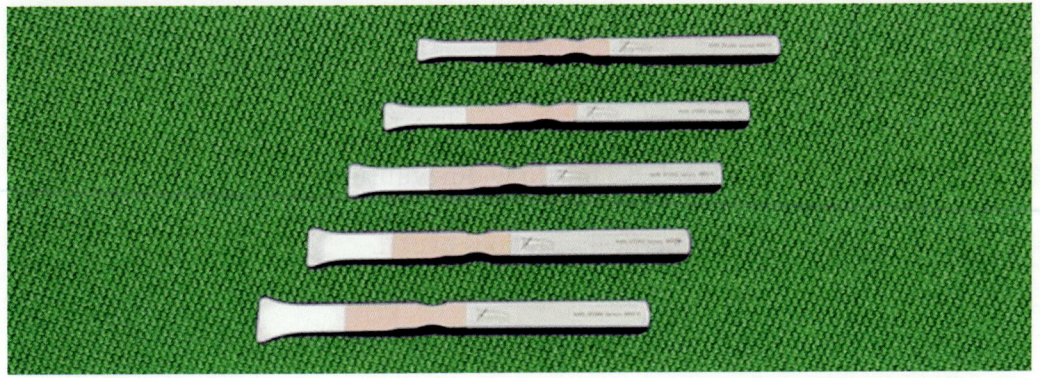

Osteotomes

Indication

- These osteotomes are specifically designed for performing nasal osteotomy.

JOSEPH RASPATORY AND GLABELLA RASPATORY

Identifying Features

- Joseph raspatory has expanded working end with horizontal and vertical serrations.
- Glabella raspatory is curved and is used in push-pull motion and is about 20 cm long.

Indication

- Surgical instrument used to smoothen and refine the edges of nasal bone and hump reduction.

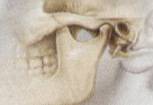

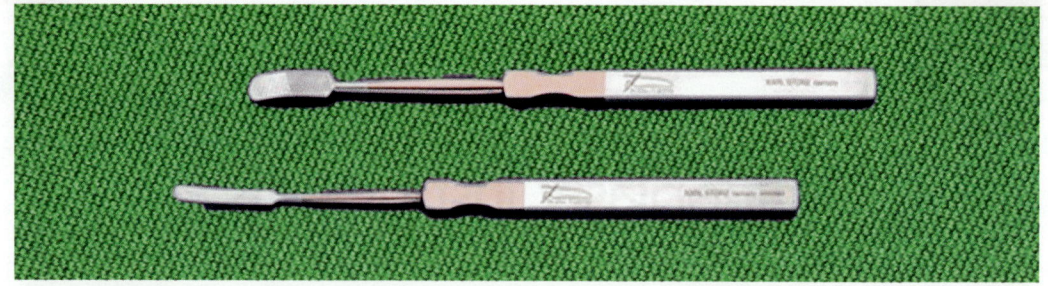

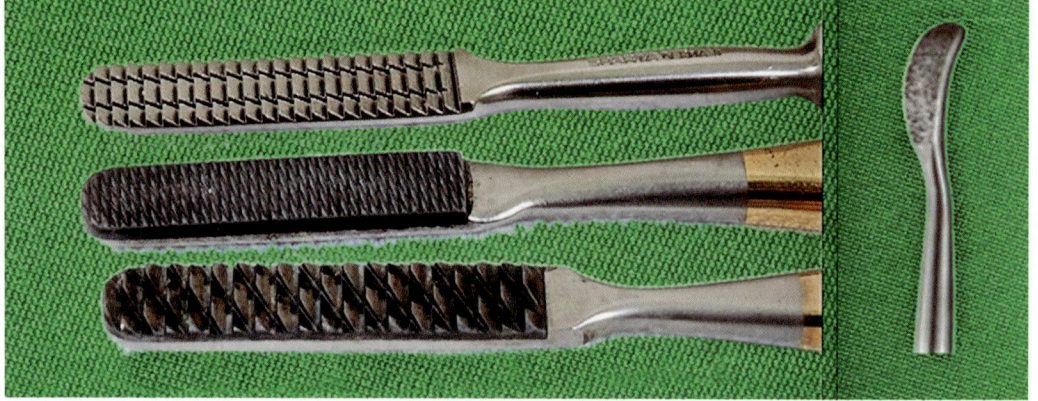

Joseph and Glabella raspatories

AUFRICHT NASAL RETRACTOR

Identifying Features

- It has a small blade which is 8.5 mm in width with angled shaft.
- Length of retractor blade is about 45 mm with pointed tip.
- The handle is broad with vertical serrations over it.

Indication

- This retractor is used for retraction of nasal skin during rhinoplasty.

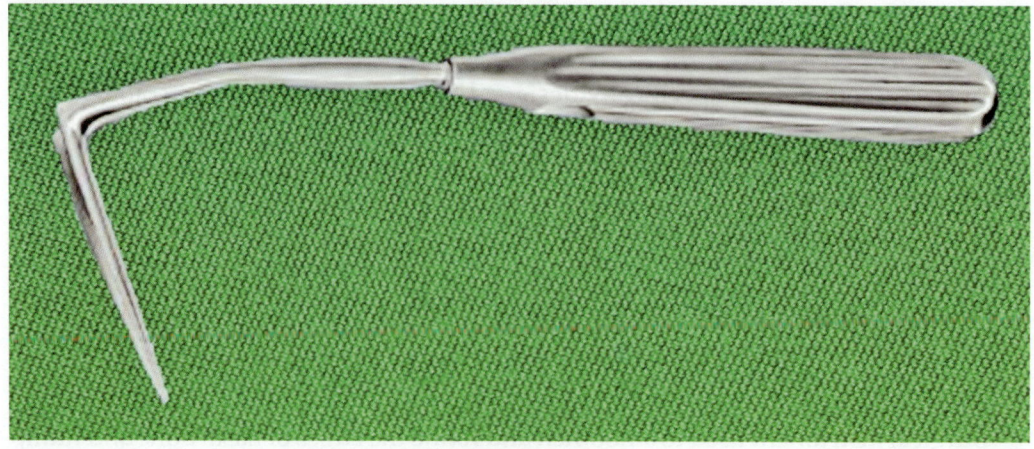

Aufricht nasal retractor

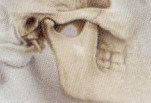
JOSEPH SKIN HOOK WITH TWO PRONGS

Identifying Features

- Joseph skin hook is a hand held retractor with two sharp prongs.
- Width is 10 mm and length is 12 mm.

Indication

- Joseph skin hook is a hand held retractor commonly used for holding back the edges of skin during intranasal (rhinoplasty) and pharyngeal procedures.

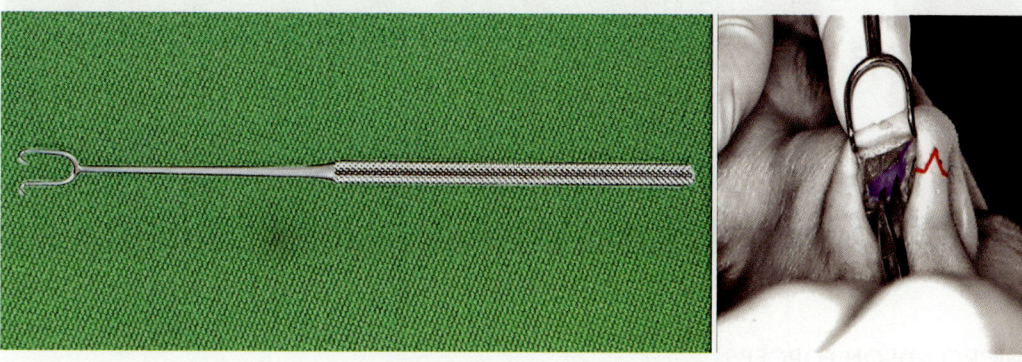

Joseph skin hook with two prongs

SKIN HOOK WITH ONE PRONG

Identifying Features

- It has very thin curved hook at the end of tool.
- The prong of the skin hook instrument can be customized to the procedure performed.
- Equipment has hook that is very sharp and thin with length of handle about 15 cm.

Indication

- A skin hook is a small instrument that is used to grasp, hold, and position delicate soft tissue during the suturing phase of surgical procedure during rhinoplasty.

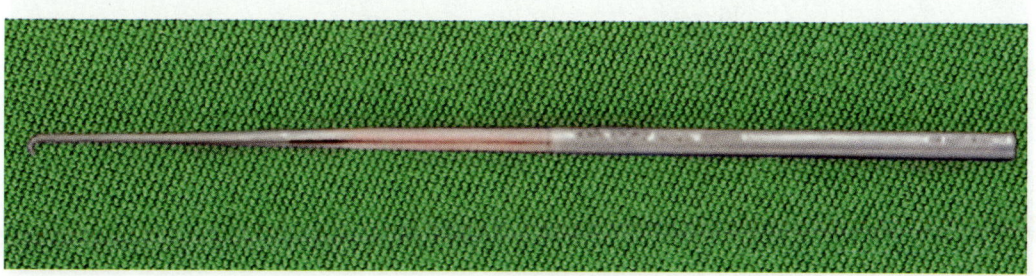

Skin hook with one prong

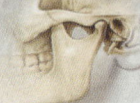

METAL MALLET

A mallet has cylindrical part which is flat on both surfaces.

Dimensions: Length 18 cm. It is similar to a hammer.

Indication

- Used for giving controlled taps on the osteotome in rhinoplasty procedure.

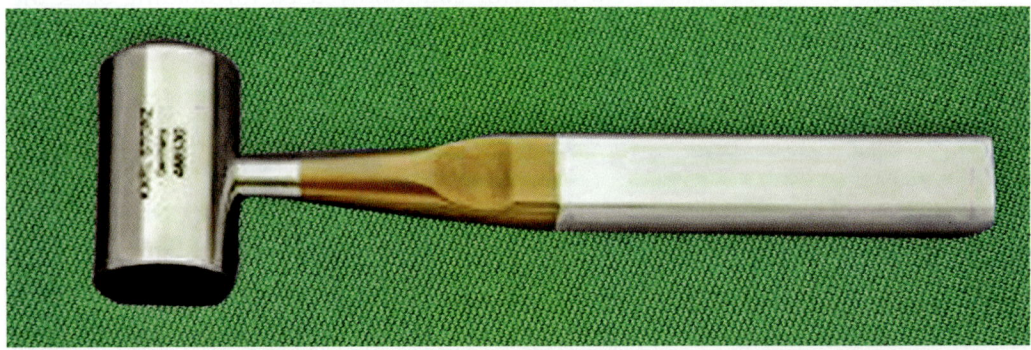

Metal mallet

MICRO ADSON FORCEPS

Delicate forceps, their tip extensions form a W-shape when held in a closed position. They are so designed that the tissues experience minimum trauma during the surgery. They are often referred to as the rat tooth forceps. Micro adson forceps is used for precise and fine handling of the soft tissue. Dimension: Length 12 cm.

Indication

- These fine delicate teeth render the Adson forceps quite adaptive for suturing the skin during cosmetic procedures and handling cartilage during rhinoplasty. With regard to nasal procedure, the Adson forceps has been shown to be particularly useful for scoring the septal cartilage during septoplasty. In addition to being useful in the correction of septum deviation it is also used for cartilage scoring in otoplasty.

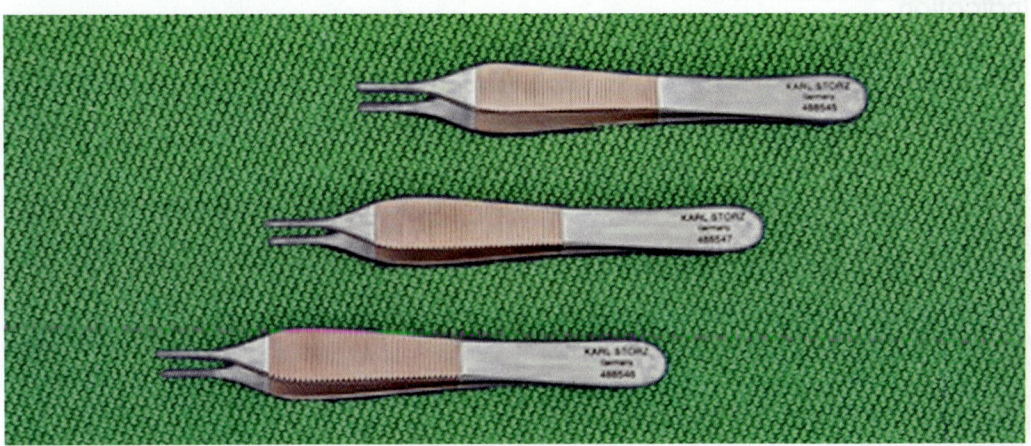

Adson forceps

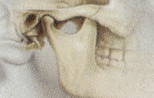
DISSECTING SCISSORS

Dissecting scissors may have curved or straight blades. Can be straight/curved, sharp and angular.

Dimension: Length 10 cm.

Indications

- Used to perform soft tissue dissection in deeper layers while doing rhinoplasty.
- Smaller sizes are used at the surface, the larger sizes used deeper in the nasal cavities.

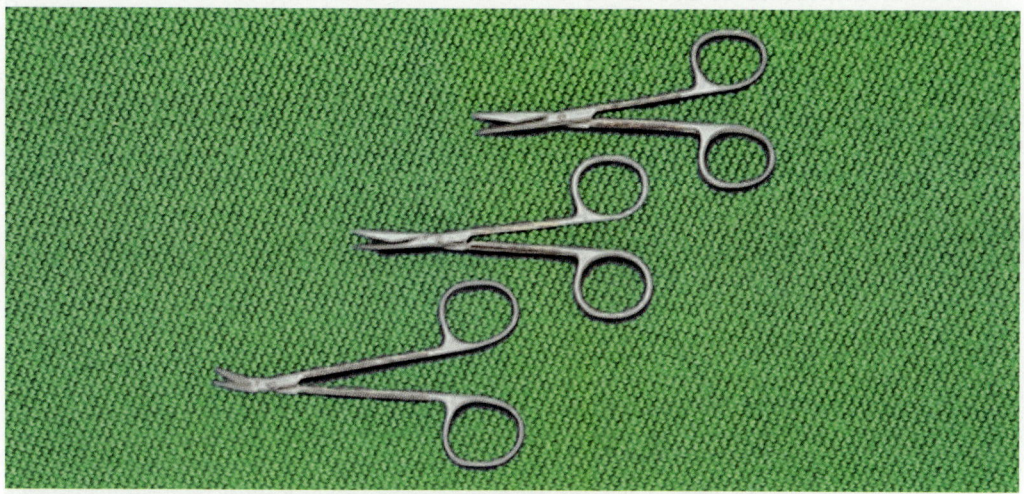

Dissecting scissors

NEEDLE HOLDER

Identifying Features

- This is a long instrument with a ratchet at non-operating end.
- The operating end has two small blades with serrations.

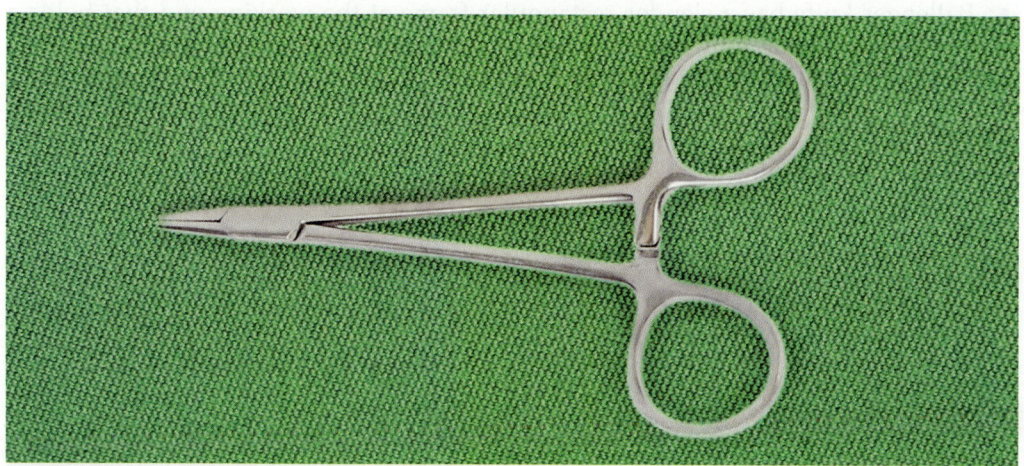

Needle holder

Indications

- The instrument is used to hold the curved needle which is used to suture the wound.
- A firm grip is essential to apply proper sutures.

GRUBER RHINOPLASTY RETRACTOR

Identifying Features

- It is plastic model of nasal architecture.

Indication

- Gruber anatomic retractor is used in the reshaping of the nose during rhinoplasty.

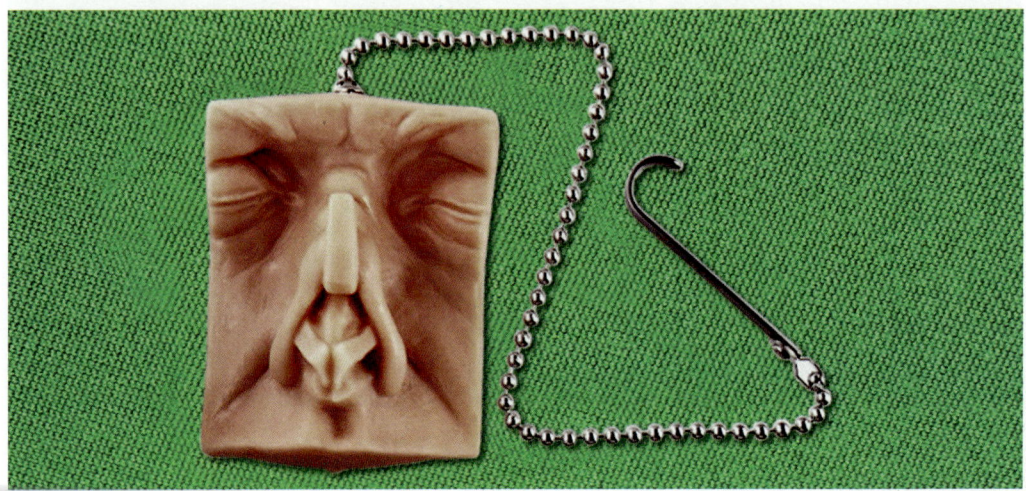

Gruber rhinoplasty retractor

BALLENGER SWIVEL KNIFE

Identifying Features

- Ballenger knife has a slender rectangular frame at the working end that holds a small blade in horizontal position between the two edges of the frame. Cylindrical working end with straight handle.

Indication

- Used to excise deformed septal cartilage enbloc, in a single movement.

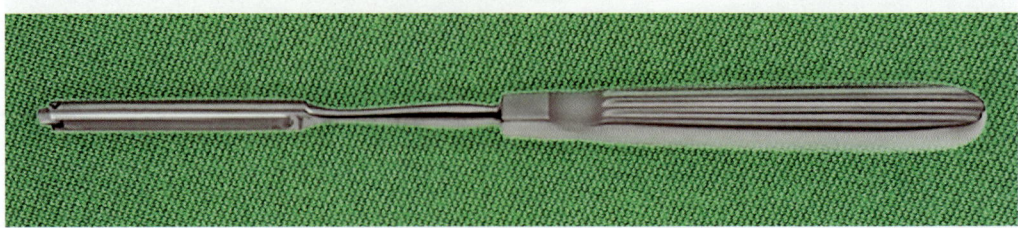

Ballenger Swivel knife

COTTLE SPECULUM

Identifying Features

- Cottle speculum is angulated narrow bladed nasal speculum.
- Handle of instruments has leaf spring with lock joint.

Indication

- Cottle nasal speculum that is introduced in between undermined tissue to achieve further separation to visualize the internal architecture of the nose during rhinoplasty procedure.

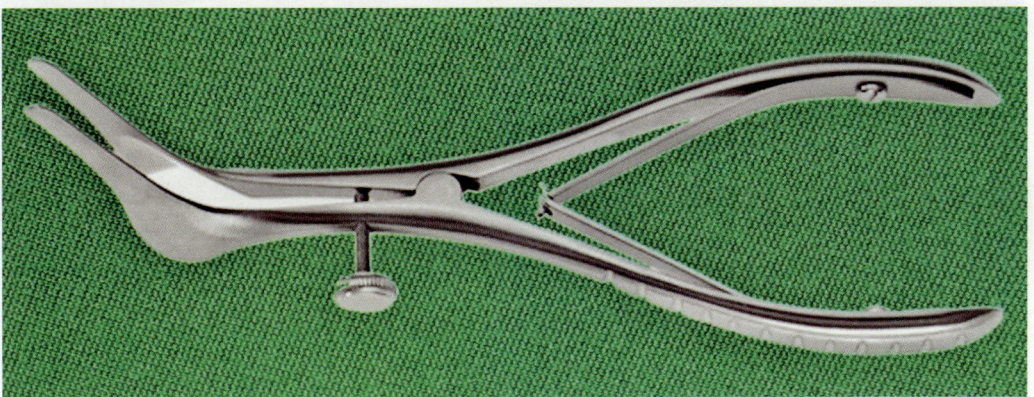

Cottle speculum

COTTLE ELEVATOR

Identifying Features

- It is a double-ended instrument, one end is sharp knife like and the other end is dull rounded.

Indications

- Cottle elevator is used for detaching overlying soft tissues from the medial cartilage.
- To raise submucosal tissue further, use of a bent dull ended elevator followed by a sharper elevator to create a submucosal tunnel until the posterior bone is reached and the bulk of the overlying tissue is raised.

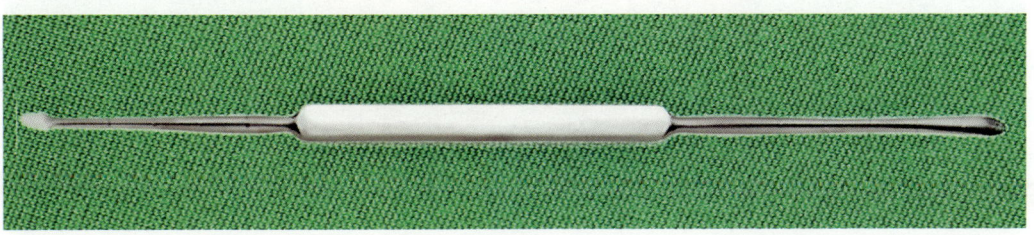

Cottle elevator

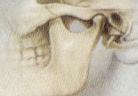

CARTILAGE FORCEP

Identifying Features

- Cartilage forceps are long with small, rectangular working end having serrations on it.

Indication

- It is used to hold the cartilage (like costal cartilage and septal cartilage) during their harvesting; for example, during augmentation rhinoplasty procedure.

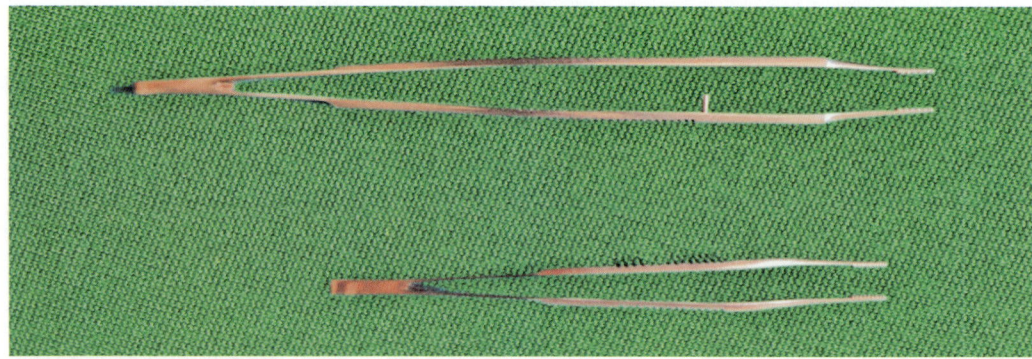

Cartilage forceps

CARTILAGE CARVING SILICON PAD

Identifying Features

- It is a flat, rectangular block made up of silicon material that can withstand with the forces applied during the cartilage carving procedure to make struts.

Indications

- It is used for carving the cartilage and designing the strut during the rhinoplasty procedure.
- It is also used during ear reconstruction in microtia cases to carve the ear framework using costal cartilage.

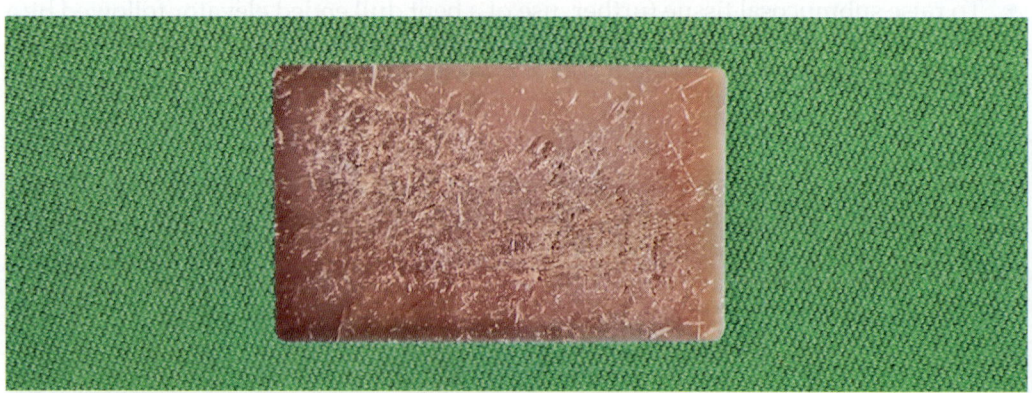

Cartilage carving silicon pad

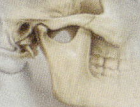

PERICHONDRIUM ELEVATOR

Identifying Features

- It is long, cylindrical with flat working end which is concave having sharp edges and rounded end. It has a large, broad handle for obtaining good grip during instrument activation.

Indications

- It is used to separate the perichondrium covering the costal cartilage during harvesting of this cartilage.
- It is used to separate the perichondrium covering the septal cartilage during the rhinoplasty procedure.

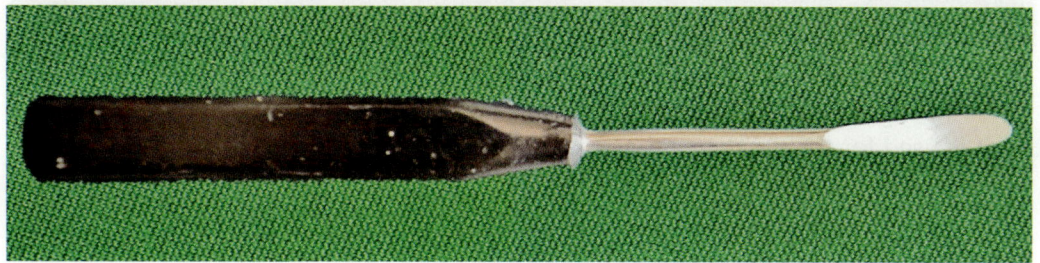

Perichondrium elevator

NASAL CHISEL WITH GUARD

Identifying Features

- It resembles a chisel except that there is a small extension present on one of the lateral edges that act as a guard, thus facilitating safe osteotomy.
- This is a paired instrument: Right and left nasal chisels with guard.

Indication

- It is used for the osteotomy of lateral nasal wall in rhinoplasty operation.

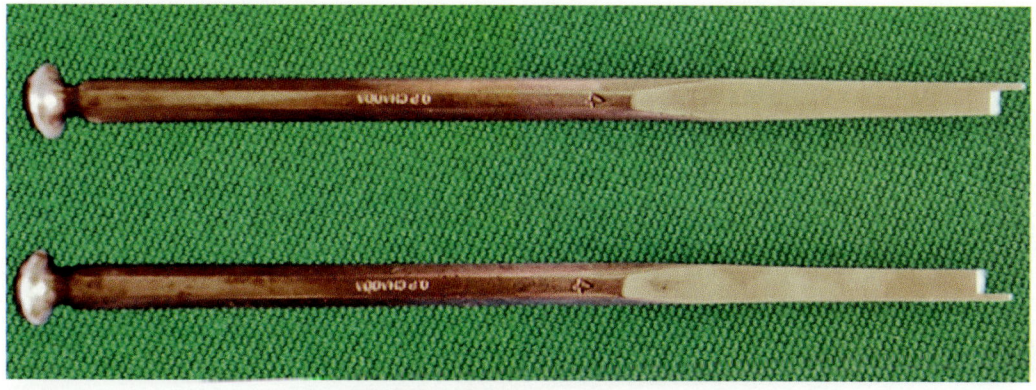

Nasal guard or lateral nasal wall osteotome

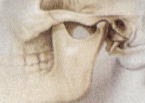

CENTRAL NASAL CHISEL

Identifying Features

- It resembles the nasal guard except that it has small extensions arising from both the edges.

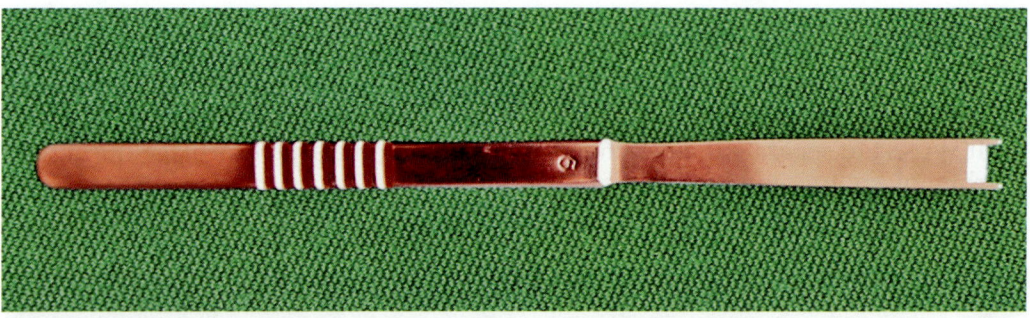

Indication

- It is used for the nasal septal osteotomy during rhinoplasty operation.

Dental Implant Instruments

Arunachaleshwar Balkunde, Swati Jadhav

IMPLANT BODY

Identifying Features

- It has 3 parts: Crest module, body, and apex.
- The coronal two-thirds of the implants have parallel walls for stability and surgical simplicity.
- Apical taper for anatomical limitations and ease surgical placement.
- Uppermost part is crest module with cylindrical smooth metal collar which transfers primary shear forces to the bone.
- The body and apex has a thread design with several parameters like thread pitch, thread shape, and thread depth.
- Available at various body diameter like 3.0 mm, 3.5 mm, 3.7 mm, 4.0 mm, 4.5 mm and 5 mm.

Indication

- It is used to restore the missing tooth.

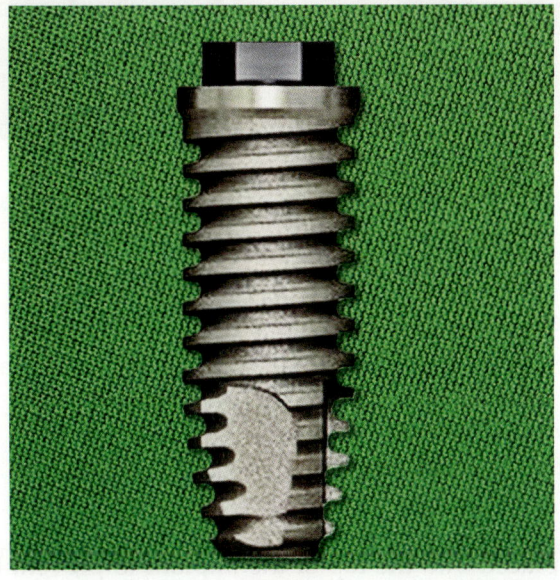

Implant body

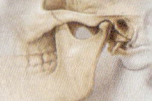

HEALING ABUTMENTS (PERMUCOSAL EXTENSION)/GINGIVAL FORMER

Identifying Features

- The 3.5 mm and 4.5 mm healing abutments are laser marked for easy intraoral identification of the prosthetic platform, emergence and height.
- Hand-tighten with the 1.25 mm hex driver.
- Healing abutments available in multiple heights to accommodate soft tissue variations, e.g. 1 mm, 2 mm and 3 mm.
- It can also be straight, flared, or anatomical.

Indication

- It is used for soft tissue healing and initial contour of the soft tissue surrounding to implant.

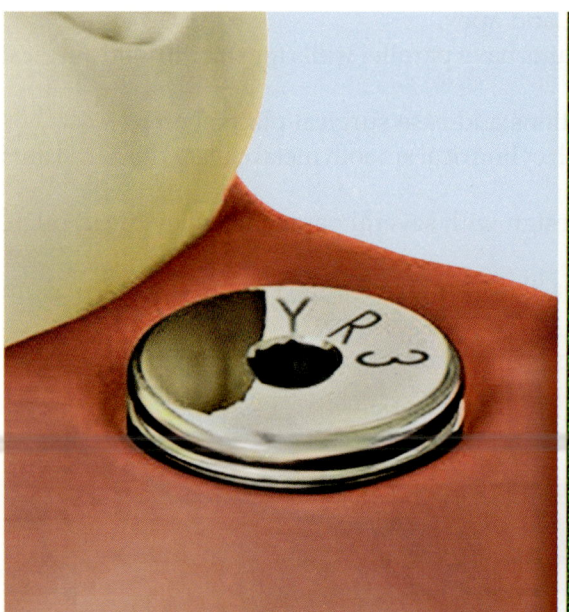
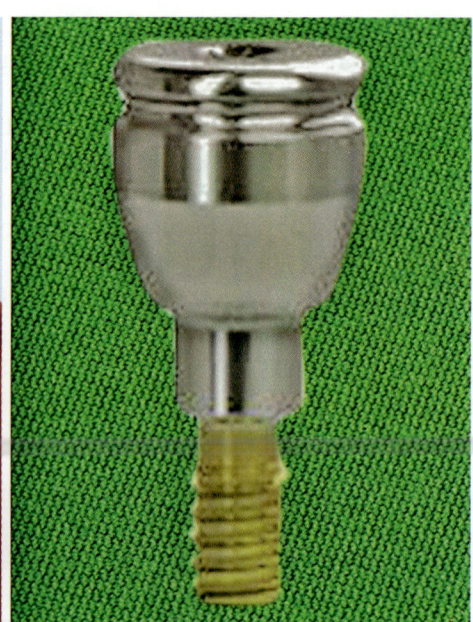

Healing abutments (permucosal extension)/gingival former

COVER SCREW

Identifying Features

- It has a cylindrical body with thread design and upper end has a cap with hexagonal slot.
- Hand-tighten with 1.25 mm hex driver.
- Color-coded for easy identification.

Indication

- Cover screw is placed into the top of the implant to prevent bone, soft tissue, or debris from invading the abutment connection area during healing.

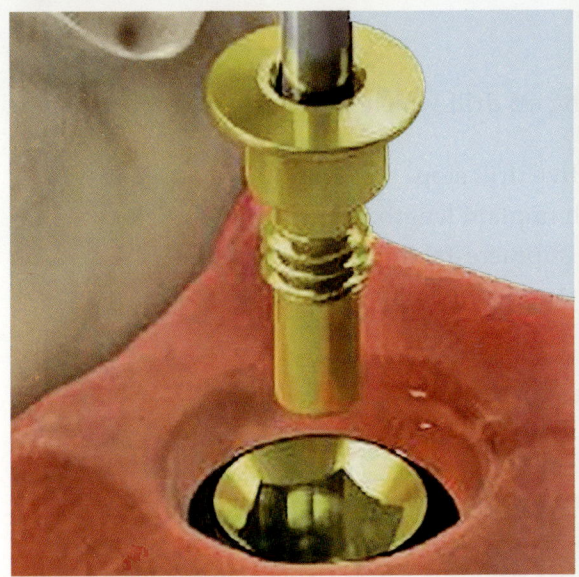
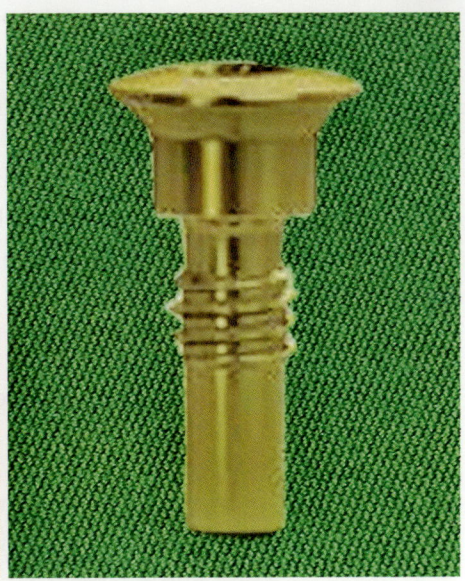

Cover screw

OSTEOTOMY DRILL (STARTER DRILL)/PILOT DRILL

Identifying Features

- 2.0 mm starter drill with chisel-tip design prevent "skating" on osseous crest.
- Starter drills having marking on drill which is 7.0 mm, 9.0 mm, 11.5 mm, 13 mm and 15 mm. It varies according to implant system.
- Prepares site for paralleling pins.
- Matte finish for increased visibility under operatory lights.

Indication

- It is used to initiate osteotomy.

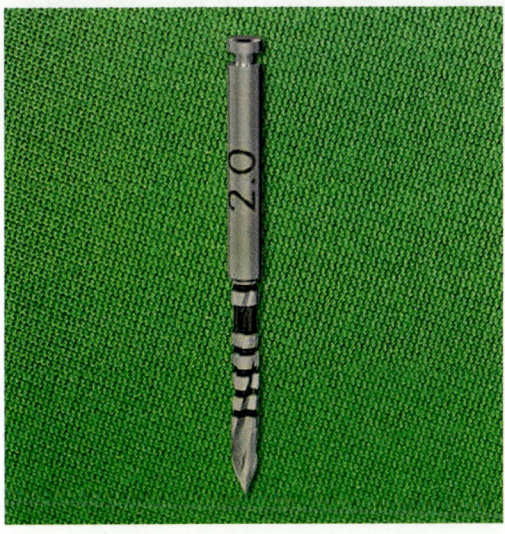

Osteotomy drill (starter drill)/pilot drill

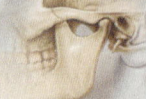

OSTEOTOMY DEPTH DRILLS WITH STOP

Identifying Features

- 2.5 mm depth drill having marking on drill which is 7.0 mm, 9.0 mm, 11.5 mm, 13 mm and 15 mm.
- Fixed circular ring acts as a definitive drill stop.
- One drill length is specific for each implant length.
- 1 mm laser-etched line guides the supracrestal implant placement.
- Matte finish for increased visibility under operatory lights.

Indication

- To set osteotomy depth when access or visibility is poor.

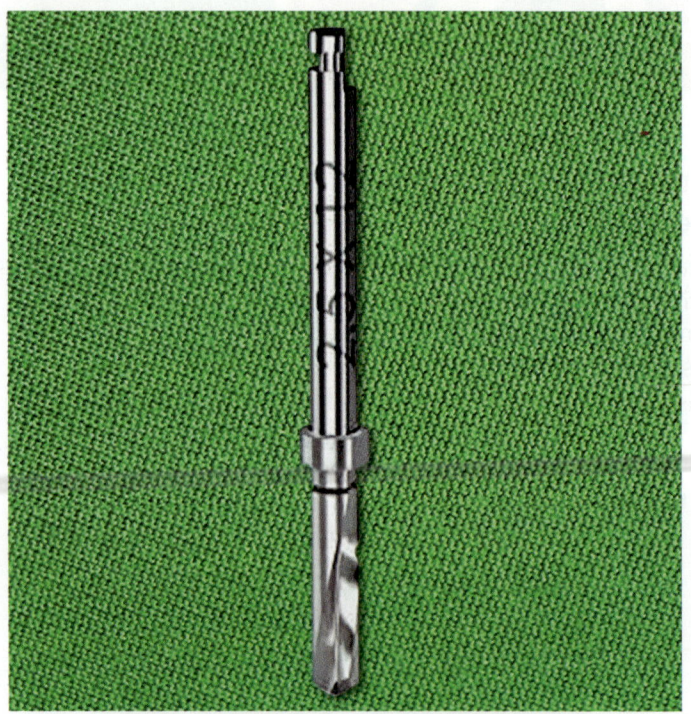

Osteotomy depth drills with stop

PARALLELING PINS

Identifying Features

- It is a smooth cylindrical pin either straight or with a 20° angle.
- It is used after 2.0 mm Starter Drill and 2.5 mm Depth Drill.
- 9 mm shank for radiographic evaluation for proximity to the adjacent anatomy.
- Hub diameter is 4.0 mm.

Indication

- To evaluate the osteotomy position and angle.

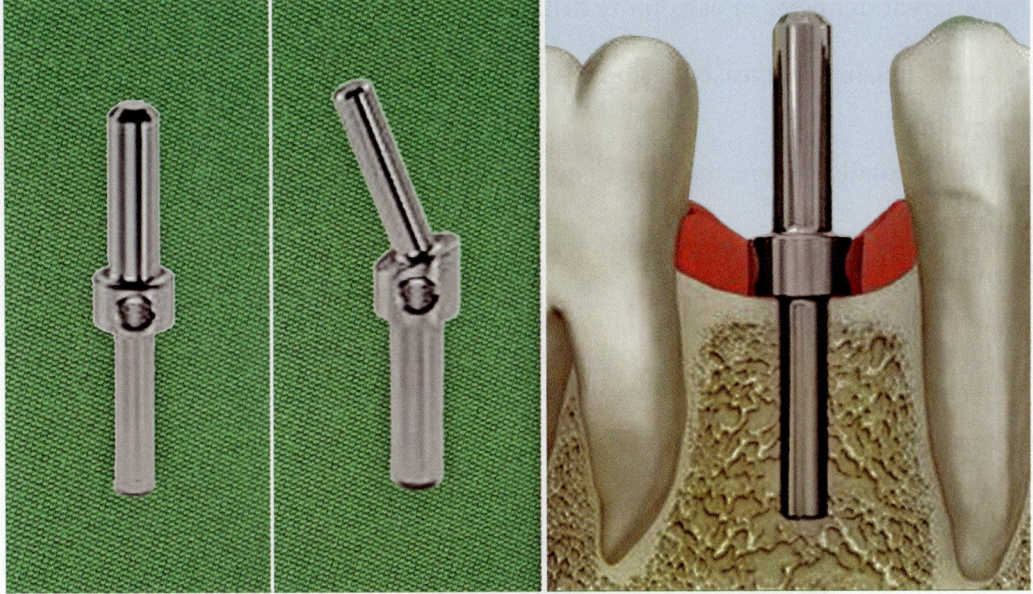

Paralleling pins

WIDTH INCREASING OSTEOTOMY DRILL

Identifying Features

- They are width increasing drills with depth, marked for reference.
- The drill tip has limited end cutting. However, the osteotomy depth can be increased with these drills as needed.

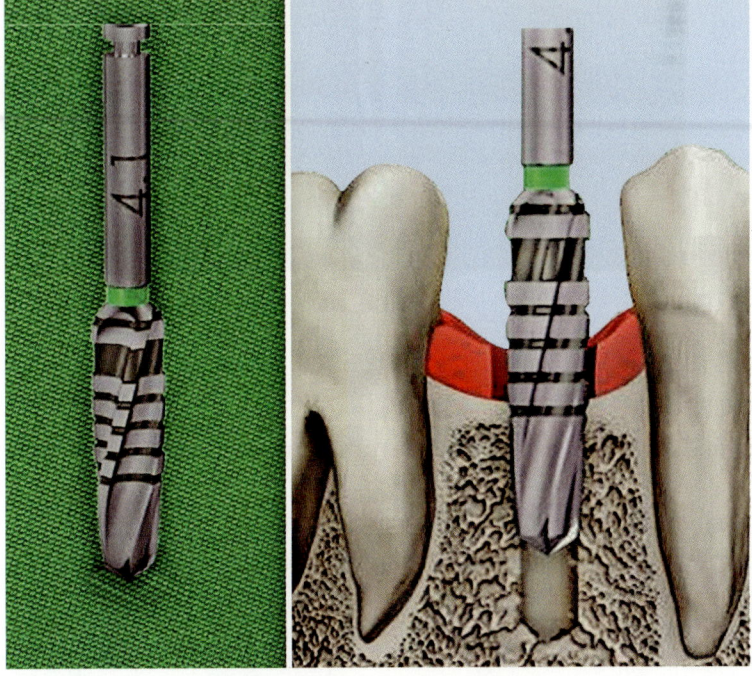

Width increasing osteotomy drill

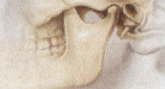

- Different diameter of osteotomy drills are 2.5 mm, 3.0 mm, 3.5 mm, 4.0 mm and 4.5 mm.
- Matte finish for increased visibility under operatory lights.

Indication

- Incrementally widens the osteotomy to reduce heat generation.

DEPTH GAUGE

Identifying Features

- Depth gauge has depth marks for reference.
- Place the depth gauge into the osteotomy site, adjust osteotomy depth as necessary.
- It is used following the final width increasing drill for each implant.

Indication

- To verify osteotomy depth.

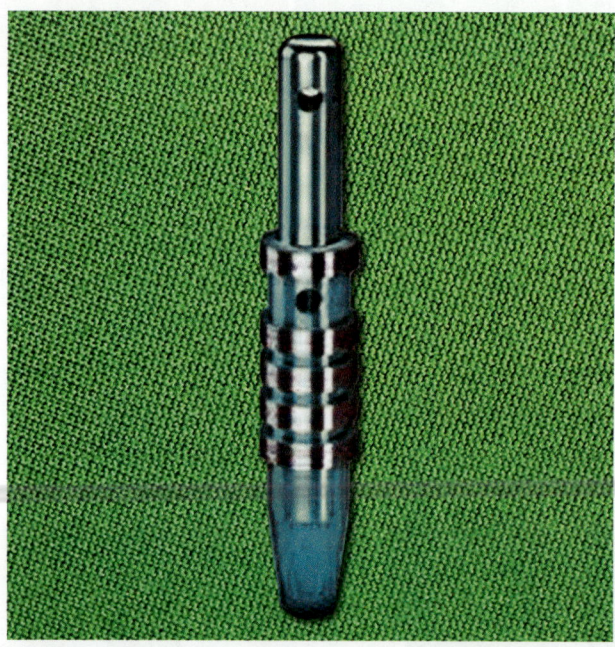

Depth gauge

CRESTAL BONE DRILLS

Identifying Features

- It is rounded and has a non-end cutting hub in the centre which is used in osteotomy.
- It is used when dense cortical bone is present at crest.
- It is used following the final width increasing drill for each implant.

Indication

- Remove cortical bone at ridge crest for pressure-free seating of the implant collar.

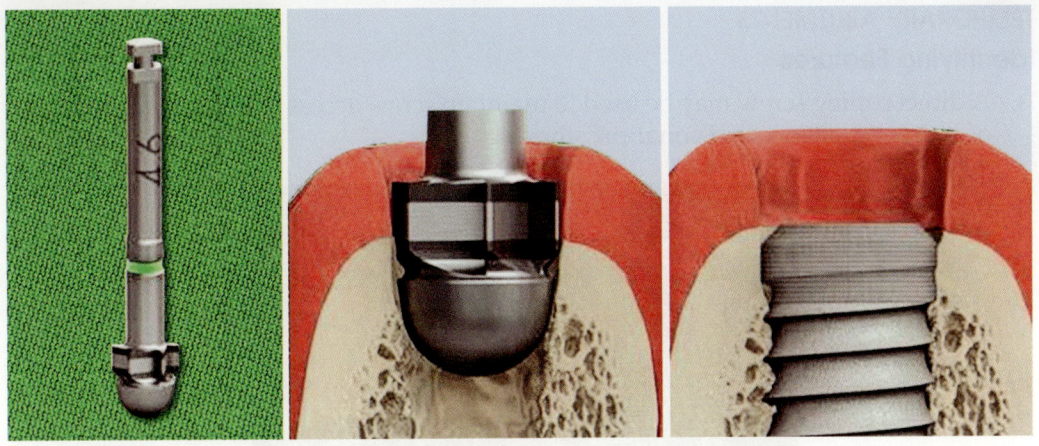

Crestal bone drills

IMPLANT DRIVERS

Identifying Features

- Implant drivers are colour coded for prosthetic connection.
- Colour coding, gray: 3.0 mm platform, yellow/green: 3.5/4.5 mm platform.

Indication

- Engage the implant's internal hex to drive and mount the implants into the osteotomy at 30 rpm or less.

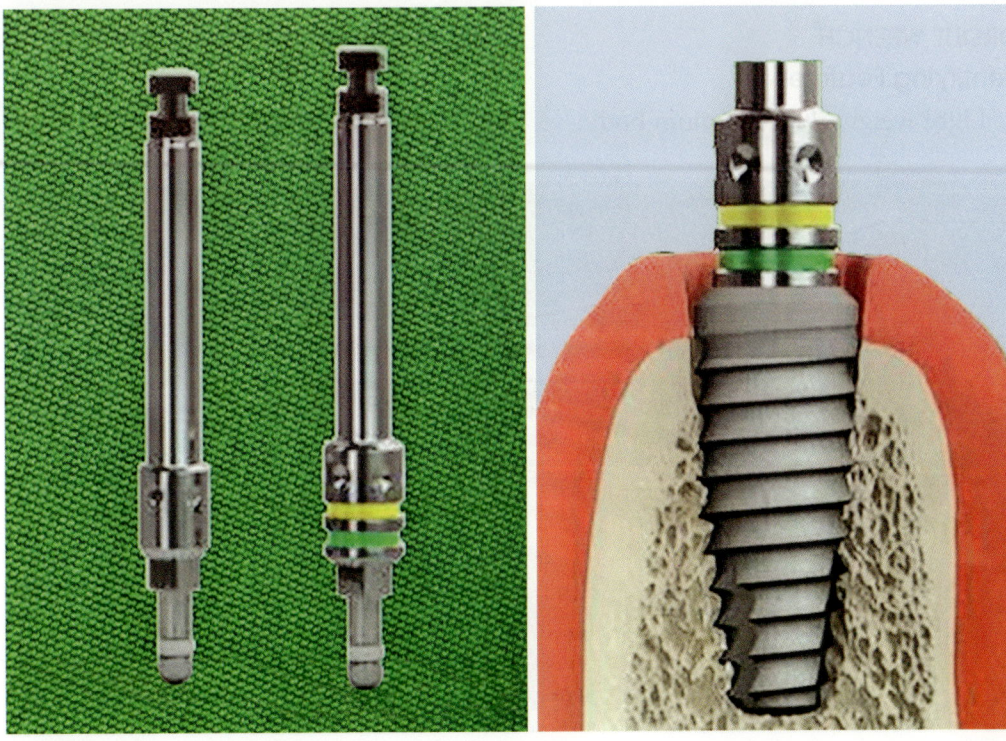

Implant drivers

TEMPORARY ABUTMENTS

Identifying Features

- A direct coping screw may be used to maintain screw access hole during fabrication of screw-retained provisional prostheses.

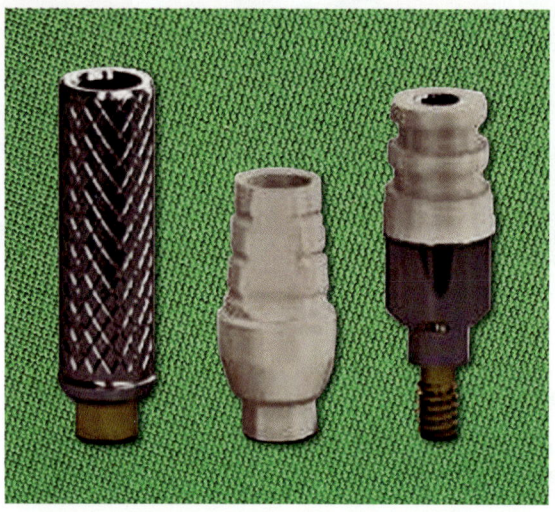

Temporary abutments

Indication

- Used for fabrication of cement- or screw-retained provisional restorations.

TORQUE WRENCH

Identifying Features

- Light weight with titanium body.

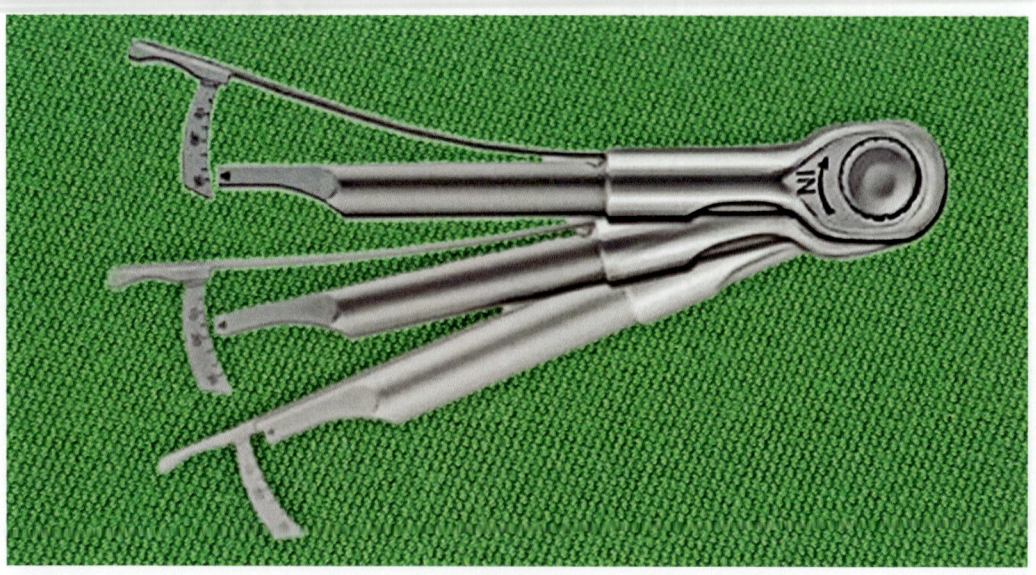

Torque wrench

- One end has calibration for torque measurement and the other end has a slot for driver to move the ratchet.

Indication

- Used to adjust the torque.

BONE PROFILERS

Identifying features

- Color-coded by prosthetic platform (gray = 3.0 mm, yellow = 3.5 mm, green = 4.5 mm).
- Profiler guide protects implant platform.

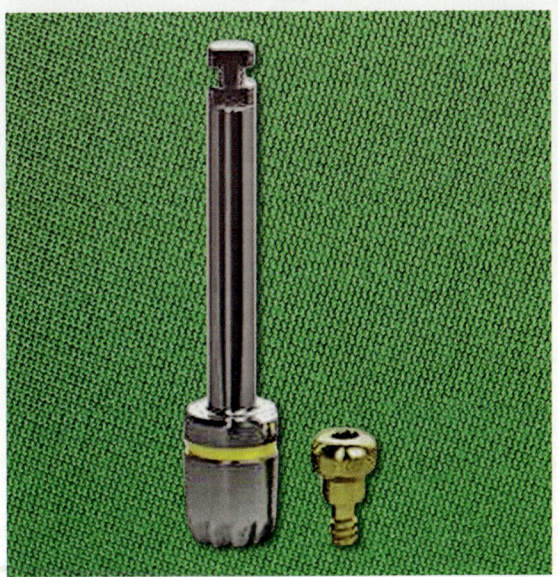

Bone profilers

Indication

- In cases where excess crestal bone has been created, use a bone profiler at implant uncovery to contour the bone. This will provide the necessary clearance for proper abutment seating.

Practice note

- Using a hex driver, remove the surgical cover cap from the implant and place the profiler guide that matches the color of the prosthetic platform. Use the profiler with copious amounts of sterile irrigation. Once the excess bone and soft tissue are removed, unscrew the guide and seat the appropriate prosthetic component.

BONE TAPS

Identifying Features

- It is site specific and used at 30 rpm or less.
- Can be driven with a hand piece, ratchet or hand wrench.
- Final instrument prior to implant placement.

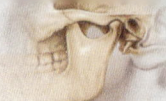

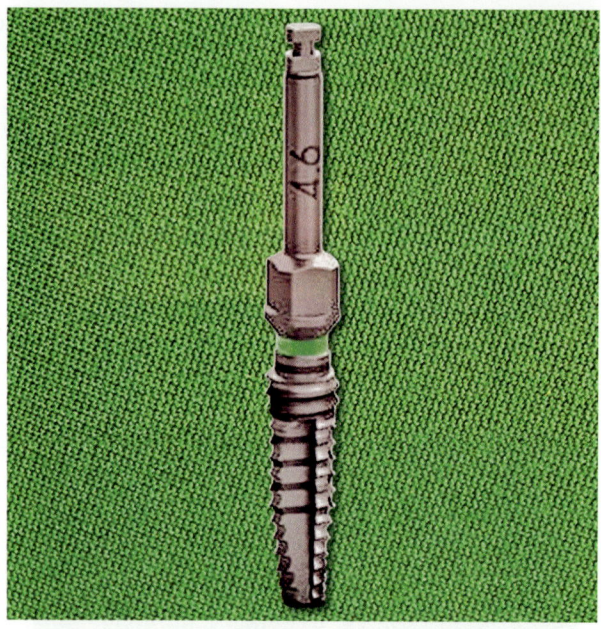

Bone taps

Indication

- To prepare dense cortical bone for implant threads.

Practice note

- Place into the osteotomy, apply firm apical pressure and rotate slowly in a clockwise direction. When the threads engage, allow the tap to feed without excessive pressure. To remove, rotate the bone tap in a counter-clockwise direction, allowing it to back out of the osteotomy. Do not pull on the bone tap to remove it from the site.

SINUS LIFT INSTRUMENTS

Indirect Sinus Lift Instruments

STRAIGHT OSTEOTOME

Identifying Features

- Straight osteotome with concave working end.
- Working end has marking at 7 mm—10 mm—11 mm—13 mm—15 mm.
- The length of osteotomes is 17.5 cm.

Types

- 2.5 , 3, 3.5, 4 and 4.5 mm diameter.

Functions

- It is used for maxillary sinus floor elevation in indirect sinus lift procedure.
- Osteotomes are used sequentially in an order like 2.5 mm, 3 mm, 3.5 mm, 4.0 mm and 4.5 mm diameter.

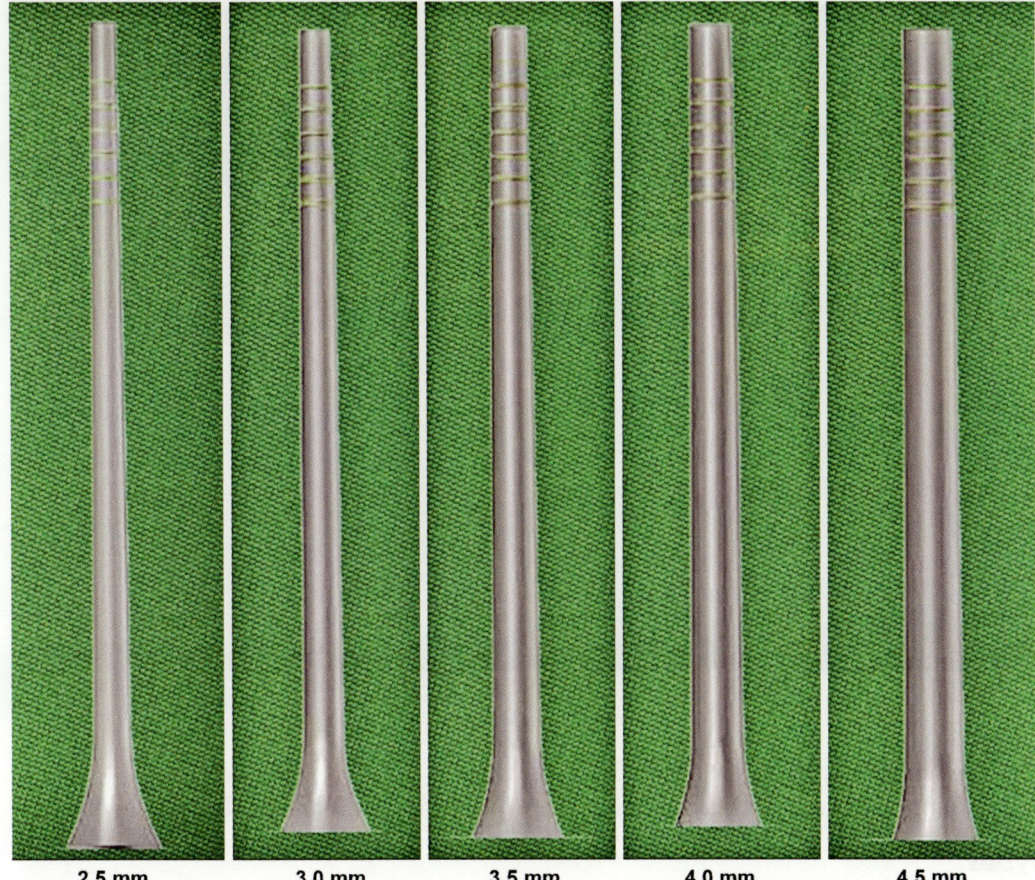

| 2.5 mm | 3.0 mm | 3.5 mm | 4.0 mm | 4.5 mm |

Straight osteotome

Practice note

- The osteotome inserted is of the same diameter as the final osteotomy.
- It is tapped firmly in 0.5 to 1.0 mm increments beyond the osteotomy until reaching its final vertical position up to 2 mm beyond the prepared osteotomy.

Indications

- It is used in SA type II bone where available bone is 10–12 mm.
- Used in sequential manner, e.g. after using pilot drill short of sinus floor, sequential osteotomes are used like 2.5 mm, 3 mm, 3.5 mm, 4 mm and 4.5 mm.
- Greenstick fractures of sinus floor should be done with larger diameter osteotomes.
- It is tapped firmly in 0.5–1 mm increments beyond the osteotomy until reaching its final position up to 2 mm beyond the prepared implant osteotomy with last diameter of osteotome.

OFFSET OSTEOTOME
Identifying Features

- Offset osteotome with concave working end.
- Working end has marking at 7 mm—10 mm—11 mm—13 mm—15 mm.

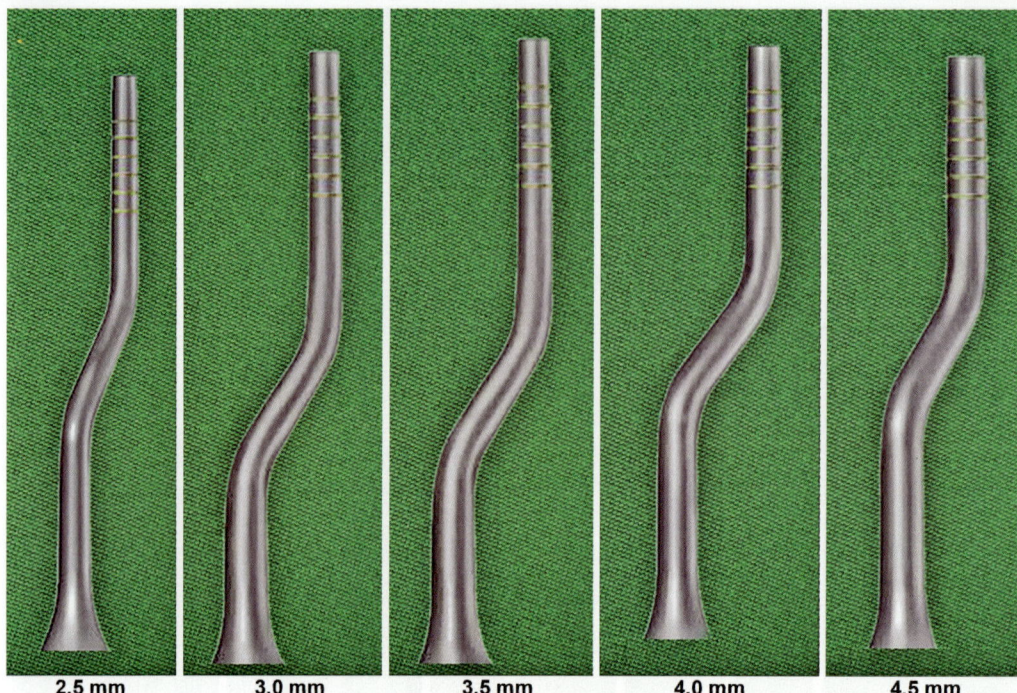

| 2.5 mm | 3.0 mm | 3.5 mm | 4.0 mm | 4.5 mm |

Offset osteotome

- The length of osteotomes is 17.5 cm.
- Different range of sizes available according to final osteotomy drills diameter.

Types

- 2.5 mm diameter
- 3 mm diameter
- 3.5 mm diameter
- 4 mm diameter
- 4.5 mm diameter

Functions

- It is used for maxillary sinus floor elevation.

Indications

- It is used in SA type II bone where available bone is 10–12 mm.
- Used in sequential manner, e.g. after using pilot drill short of sinus floor, sequential osteotome are used like 2 mm, 2.5 mm, 3 mm, 3.5 mm and 4 mm, greenstick fractures of sinus floor should be done with larger diameter osteotomes.
- Osteotome is tapped firmly in 0.5–1 mm increments beyond the osteotomy until reaching its final position up to 2 mm beyond the prepared implants osteotomy.

Practice note

- The osteotome inserted is of the same diameter as the final osteotomy is selected.

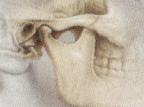
SINUS LIFT CURETTE

Identifying Features

- It is short-bladed soft tissue curette with right angle and bends at both working ends.
- Working end with curved and sharp blade.
- The length of curette is 18 cm.
- Various designs of curette available with small and large size.

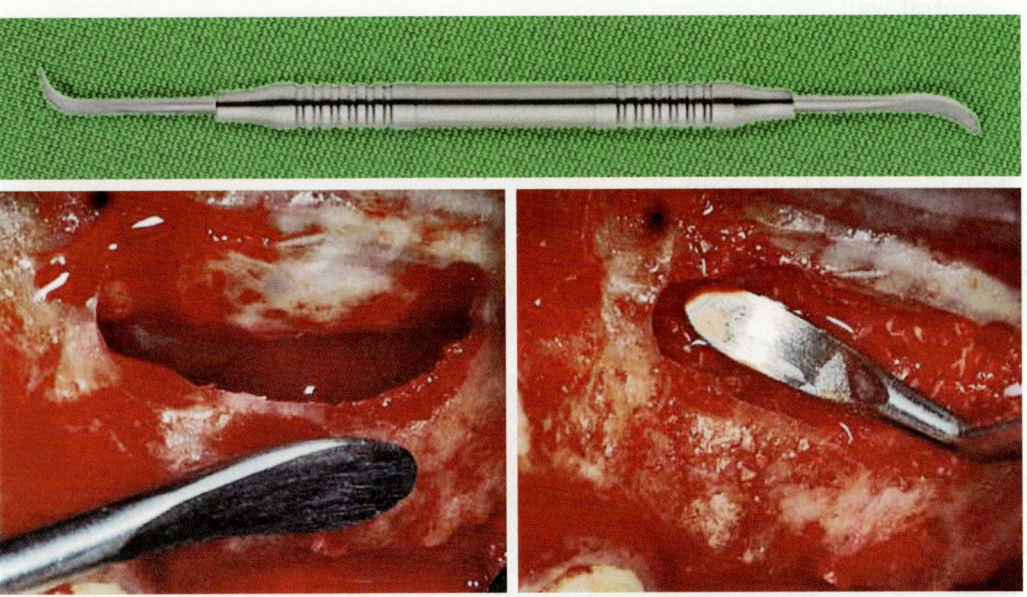

| Lateral access window | Soft tissue curette membrane elevation |

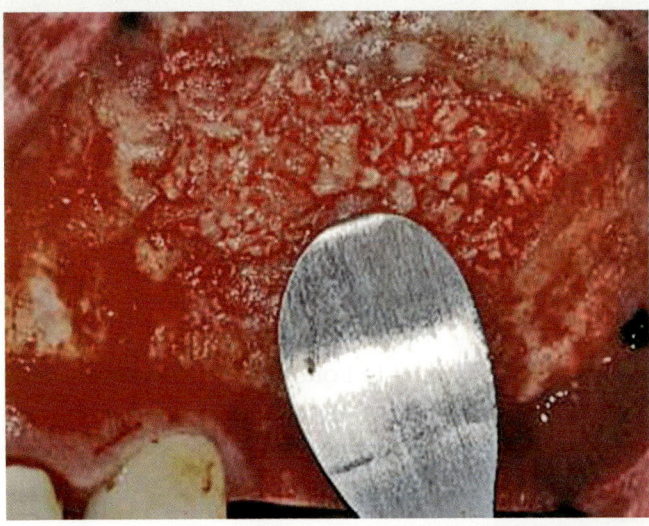

Autogenous bone graft

Sinus lift curette

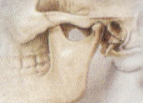

Indication

- It is used to release of the sinus membrane from the surrounding walls of the sinus without tearing from the sharp bony access margins.

Practice note

- The curved portion is placed against the window, whereas the sharp edge is placed between the sinus membrane and the margins of the inner wall of the antrum for a depth of 2 to 4 mm. The curette is slide along the bone margins, 360° around the access window. It leads to elevation of sinus membrane from antral wall.

BONE CARRIERS

Identifying Features

- It has 3 circular attachment, one at end and two at side of central body.
- It has central hollow tube.

Indication

- It is used as bone carrier to the osteotomy site.

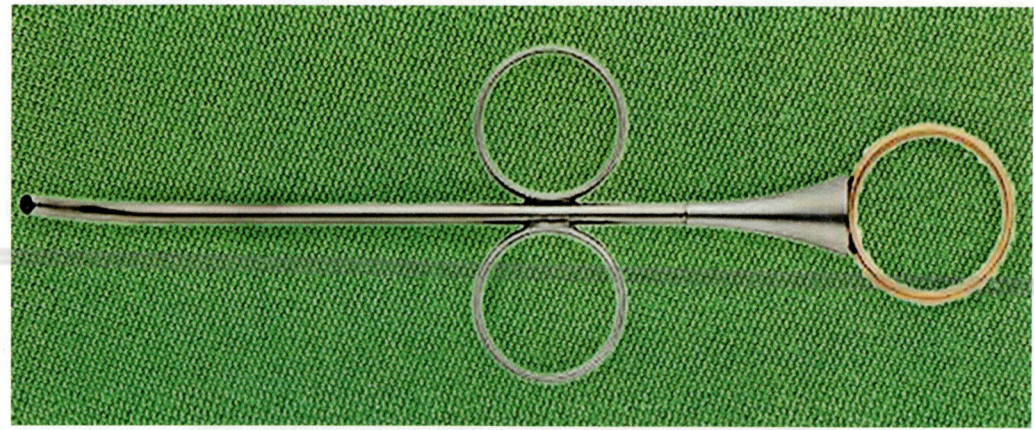

Bone carriers

BONE MORSELIZER

Identifying Features

- It is forceps type where working end has two slots, one for bone placement and the other to crush the bone.
- The working end also has a key to bone placement slot with mesh-like titanium inside the slot and flat disk on the other end.
- While tightening the key leads both slot to come together and crush the autogenous bone graft.

Indication

- It is used to mill the autogenous small and medium size bone graft.

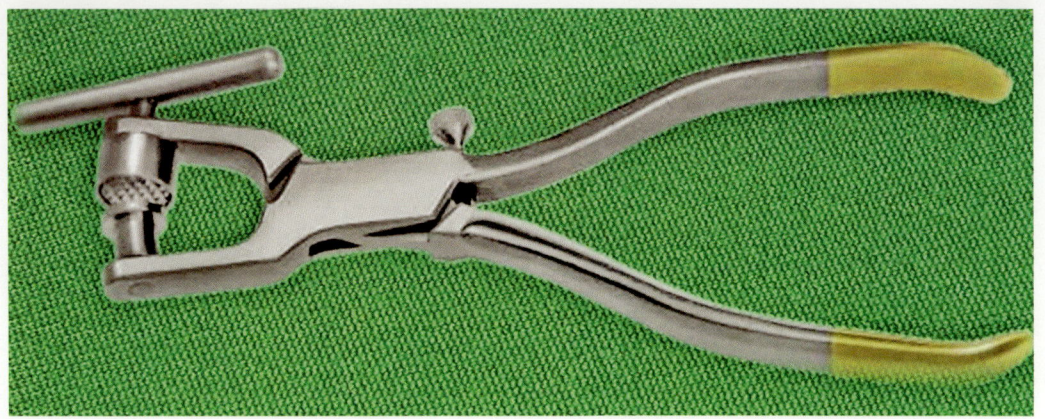

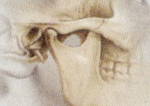

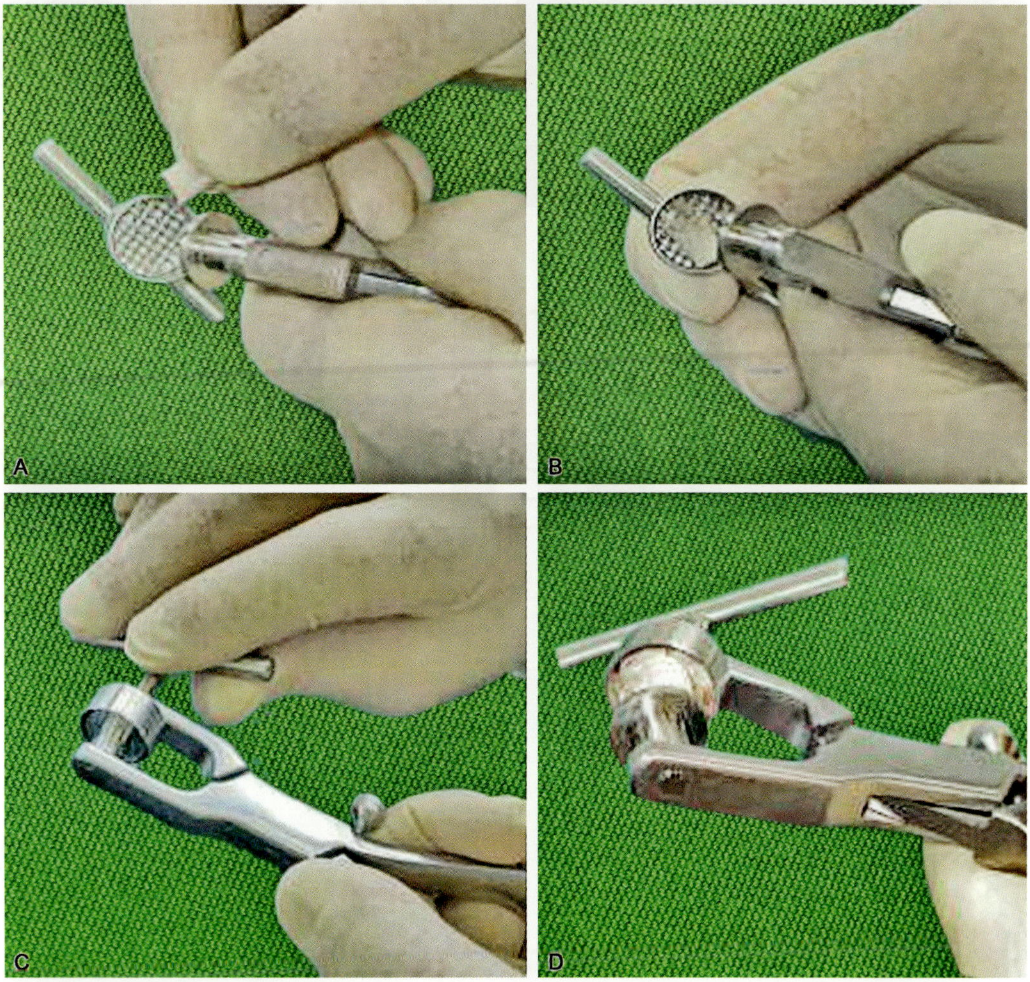

Bone morselizer

BONE SPREADER KIT

Identifying Features

- It has pointed tip and it increases in diameter from tip to handle.
- Comes in different sizes from 2.5 mm, 3 mm, 3.5 mm, 4 mm and 4.5 mm

Indications

- It is used for alveolar bone expansion in narrow ridge cases.
- Used in D3 and D4 kind of bone.

How to use?

- Make a initial hole with 2 mm drill.
- Expand the hole using the instruments of desired size.

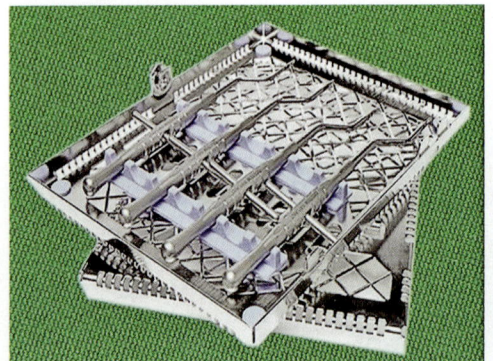 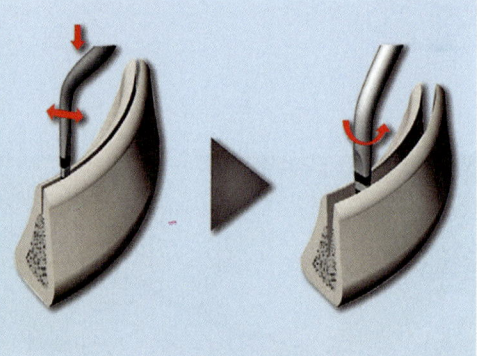

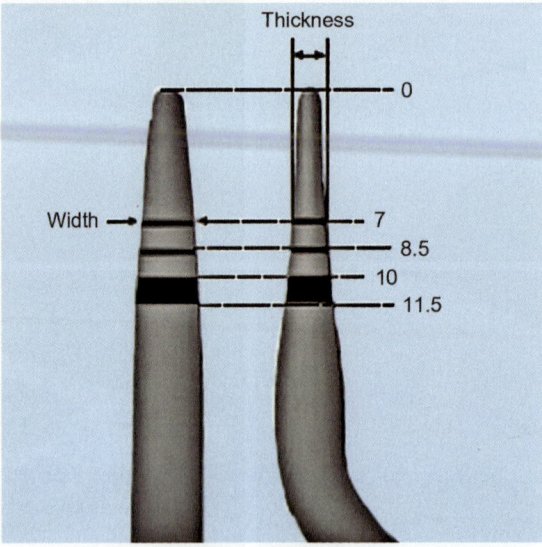

Bone spreader kit

RIDGE SPLIT AND RIDGE EXPANSION KIT

Contents of Ridge Split Kit

- Osteoplasty drill
- Disc saw
- Pilot drill

- Bone spreading drill in sequence of 2.5 mm, 3 mm, 3.5 mm, 4.0 mm and 4.5 mm
- Chisels

Indications for Ridge Split

- Used only in ridge width deficiency.
- Minimum ridge width (3.0 mm).
- Adequate available bone height (10 mm).
- No vertical ridge defects or severe concavities should be present.

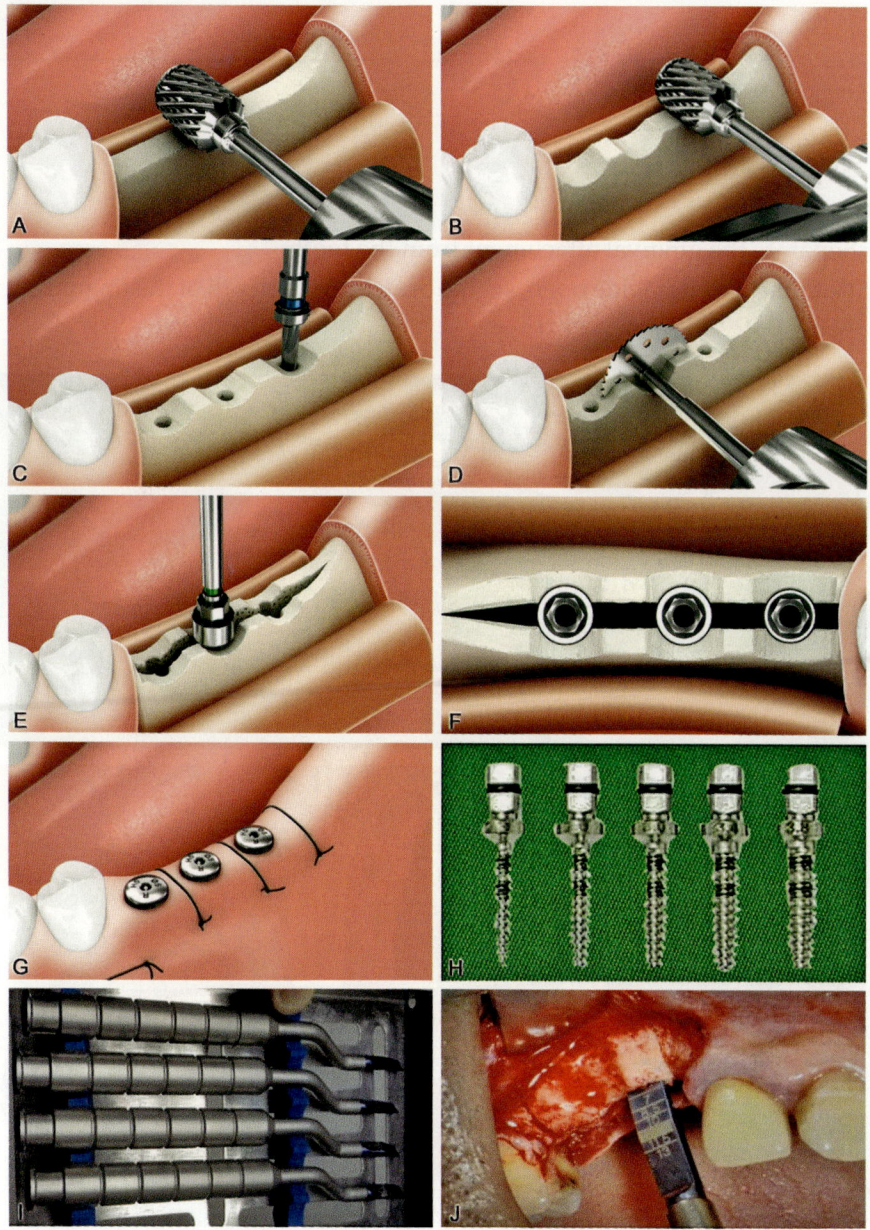

Ridge split kit, A. Osteoplasty with crest remover drill; B. Used for indentation of implant position, C. Use of pilot drill to full depth; D. Vertical sawing and horizontal sawing; E. Drills used for bone expansion and self tapping; F. Implants in position; G. Closure; H. Bone spreading drill; I. Chisels; J. Ridge split with chisels

Advanced Instruments in Oral and Maxillofacial Surgery

Ashish Satpute, Shraddha Patil, Shameen Sultana

PHYSICS FORCEPS

How to use?

Step 1: Separate the gingival attachment from the tooth

Step 2: With the handles wide open, set the beak into the depth of the lingual or palatal sulcus on solid root surface.

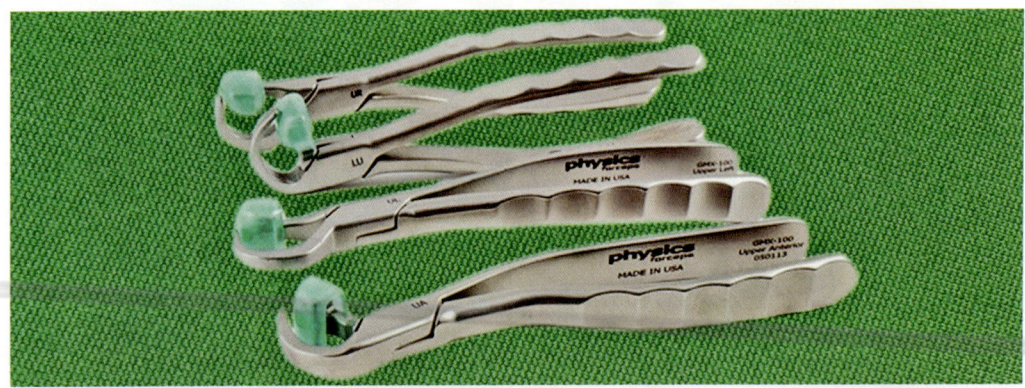

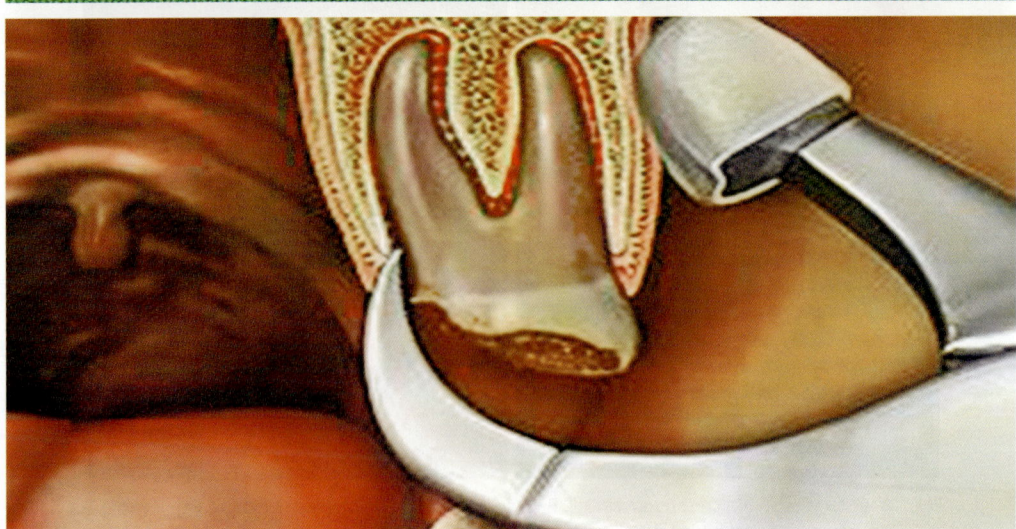

Physics forceps

Step 3: Set the bumper perpendicular to the tooth at about the level of the mucogingival junction.

Note: The greater the distance between the beak and the bumper, the greater the arc of rotation, consequently achieving vertical lift.

Step 4: Without squeezing the handles or moving your arm, begin to apply a steady, very slow rotational force in the direction of the bumper.

Step 5: The buccal rotation of the tooth and vertical lift is successful by rotating your wrist only. You will soon feel the tooth move and slightly elevate occlusally from the socket. Stop rotating at this point.

Step 6: Initially, you may want to avoid unnecessary damage to the buccal plate by not proceeding with the physics forceps beyond the first sign of the tooth "popping" loose. If the tooth has not elevated sufficiently to grasp it with your fingers, consider using a hemostat, ronguers or conventional forceps to lift it out.

Indications

- Using the physics forceps it is possible to perform difficult extractions (such as retained roots and endodontically treated teeth) in 1–2 minutes or less. In most cases it is not even necessary to reflect a flap.
- Use the physics forceps to loosen teeth, not to remove them. Wrist action is critical and twisting and rotating the root is not needed or recommended.
- Depending on the patient's anatomy and degree of eruption, the physics forceps can occasionally be used on 3rd molars; however, there is a set of forceps specifically designed to remove third molars.

POWERED PERIOTOMES

Periotomes are extraction instruments that employ the mechanisms of "wedging" and "severing" to facilitate tooth removal. Periotomes are composed of very thin metallic blades that are gently wedged down the periodontal ligament (PDL) space in a repetitive circumferential fashion. In addition to minimally invasive luxation, the periotome blade severe sharpey's fibers that secure the tooth within the socket. Once a

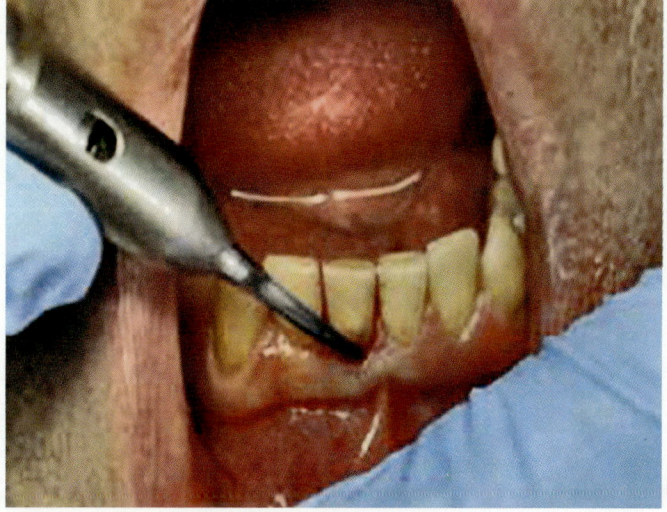

Powered periotomes

majority of sharpey's fibers have been separated from the root surface, rotational movements allow for extraction of the tooth with minimal lateral pressure. This reduces potential trauma to adjacent bone and associated gingival structures.

Disadvantage

Disadvantages of the periotome include provider fatigue and adding a significant amount of time to the extraction procedure.

How to use?

- The Powertome combines the atraumatic extraction and advantages of the periotome with mechanized speed.
- The Powertome is an electric unit that has a handpiece with a periotome blade that is controlled by a foot switch.
- The automated periotome blade is controlled by a solenoid within the handpiece.
- Power output to the handpiece is regulated by the controller box and may be adjusted to 10 different power settings.
- The Powertome is operated by selecting a power setting on the controller unit and inserting the blade into the PDL space.

INSTRUMENTS USED FOR INCISION AND CLOSURE

LASERS

Laser is often ideally suited for excisional biopsy. Vessels larger than the zone of thermal coagulation (about 500 microns for the carbon dioxide laser) will still bleed and will need to be ligated or electrocoagulated. As opposed to incisional biopsy, when performing excisional biopsy, greater consideration must be given toward protecting adjacent vital structures. Although the laser is often a better or even an ideal tool for protecting nearby anatomic structure, judiciousness should be exercised near ducts, vessels, nerves commissures, teeth and bone.

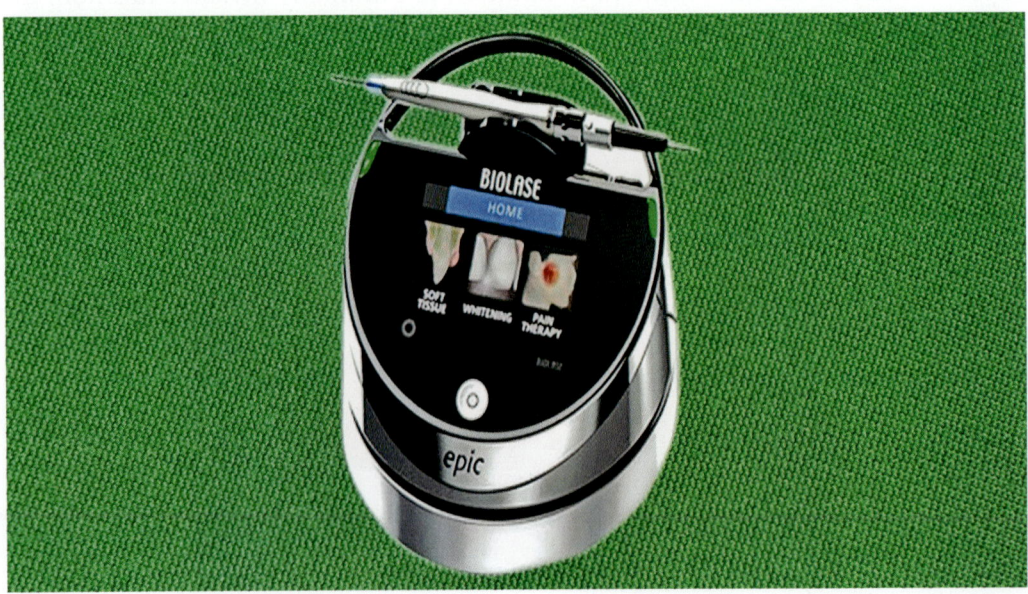

Laser system

Types of Lasers

1. Argon
2. Diode
3. Neodynium: YAG
4. Holmium: YAG
5. The Erbium family
6. CO_2

Indications

- Incisional biopsy technique.
- Excisional biopsy technique.
- Cosmetic and facial dermatologic uses of the laser include the following:
  - Lentigines
  - Seborrheic keratosis
  - Superficial pigmentation
  - Solar keratosis
  - Skin wrinkles
  - Blepharoplasty
  - Endoscopic brow lift
  - Scar revision
  - Melasma.

SKIN STAPLES

Indication

The skin staple is a medical device that places metal staples across the skin edges to bring the skin together. The area must be anesthetized before placing the staples. The main advantage of staples over sutures is that they can be placed quickly. Speed may be an important advantage when you need to close a bleeding wound quickly (e.g. on the scalp) to decrease blood loss. Its disadvantages are staples tend to leave more noticeable marks in the skin compared with sutures. They should not be used on the face.

Technique

1. The edges must be everted. Usually an assistant must help by using forceps to hold the skin edges so that the dermis on each side touches.
2. Place the center of the stapler (usually an arrow on the stapler marks the center) at the point where the skin edges come together.
3. Gently touch the stapler to the skin; you do not have to push it into the skin. Then grasp the handle to compress it; the compression releases the staple.
4. Release the handle, and move the stapler a few millimeters back to separate the staple from the stapling device.
5. The staples should be placed about 1 cm apart.

To Remove the Staples

A staple remover device can be used to remove the staples easily. Put the jaws under the staple, and close the device. This bends the staple and allows it to be removed.

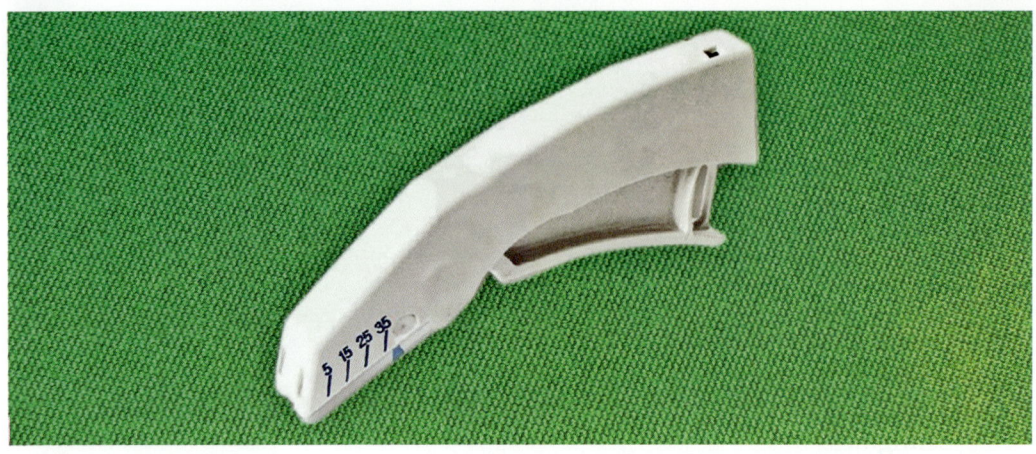

Skin staples

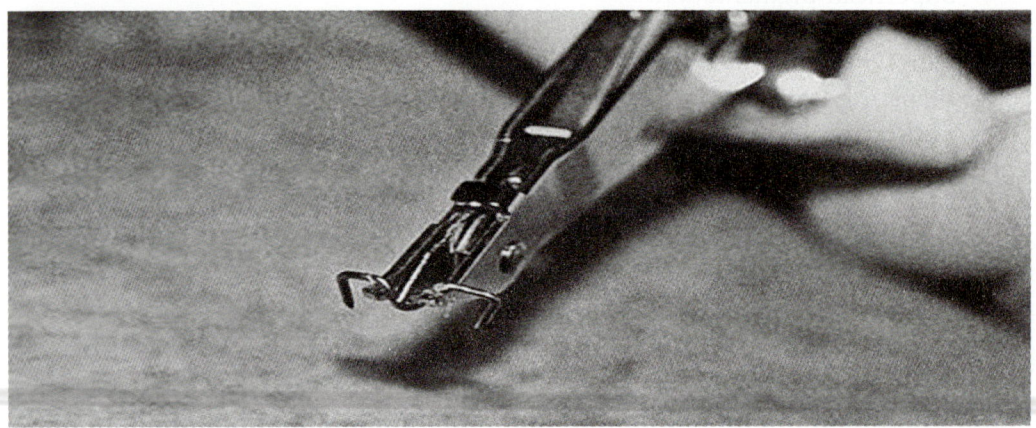

Skin staple remover

If you do not have a staple remover, a clamp can be placed under the staple. Then open the clamp to bend the staple so that it can be removed.

Removing a staple in this fashion can be painful.

INSTRUMENTS USED FOR MINIMALLY INVASIVE SURGICAL TECHNIQUE

ENDOSCOPIC INSTRUMENTS

- Endoscopes are minimally invasive diagnostic medical instruments used to evaluate interior surface of an organ. An endoscope is a flexible tube equipped with lenses and a light source. Illumination is done by the help of a number of optical fibers. Video endoscopy performed by attaching in microchip camera at the insertion tube, setup image is viewed on a video monitor.

Equipment

- A 4 mm diameter 30° angle scope (Karl Storz, Germany), a 4 mm endoscope mounted retractor (Isse Dissector Retractor, Karl Storz, Germany), which maintains the optical cavity, and a video system (Olympus America, Lake Success, New York) to project the endoscopic image onto a monitor display.

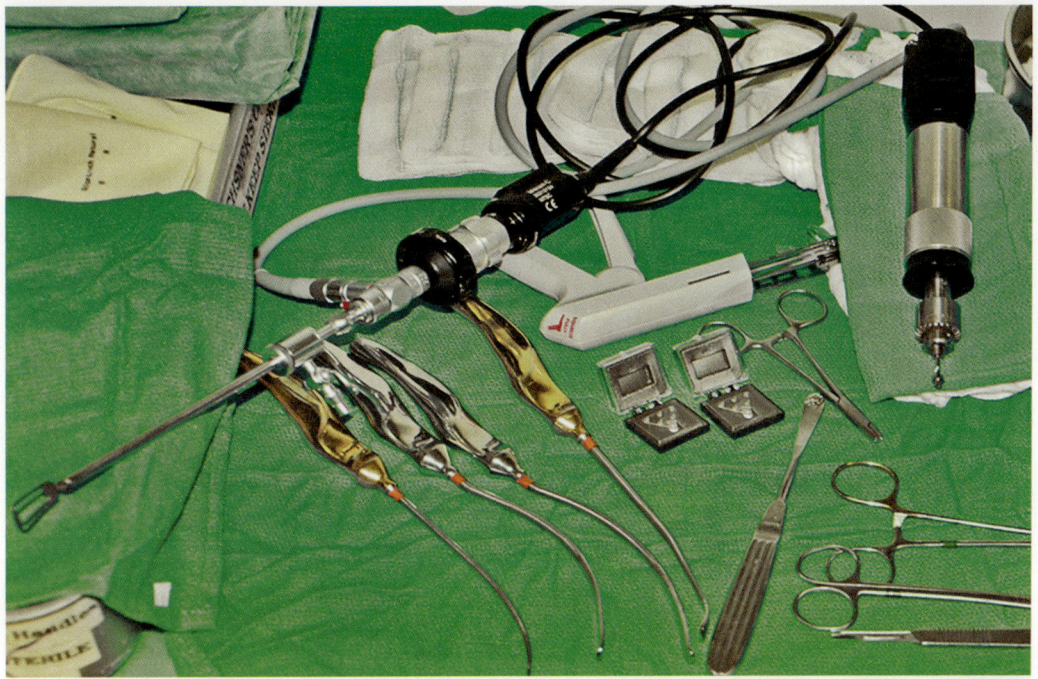

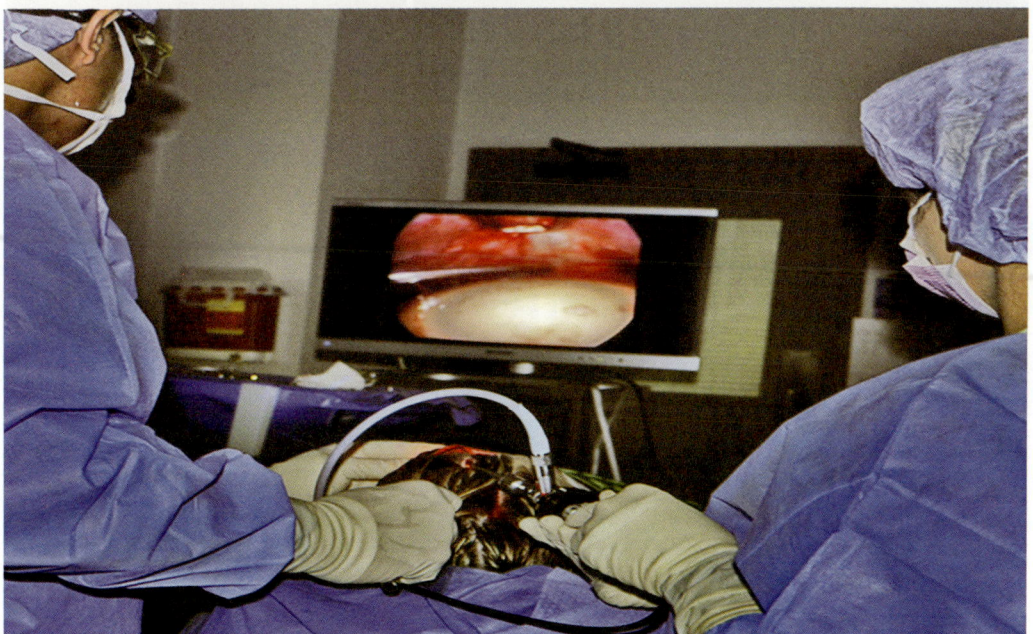

Endoscopic instruments, 30° endoscope, endotine setup

Indications

- The endoscopic approach described here has the potential to reduce morbidity by limiting scars, reducing the risk to the facial nerve, and eliminating the need for MMF, all while embracing the accepted advantages of anatomic reduction and rigid fixation.

- The decrease in morbidity associated with the endoscopic approach may expand the indications for reduction and rigid fixation in the future.

PIEZOSURGERY UNIT

Piezosurgery uses modulated ultrasonic vibration that allows controlled cutting of bony structures. Delicate bone can be cut efficiently with great precision without destructing soft tissues.

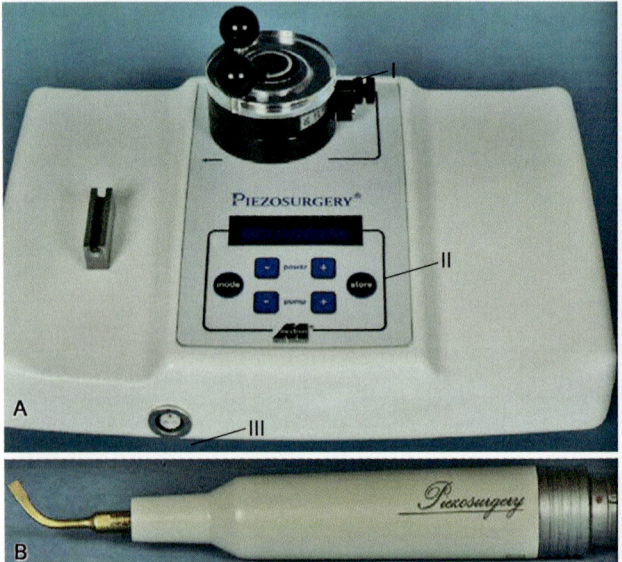

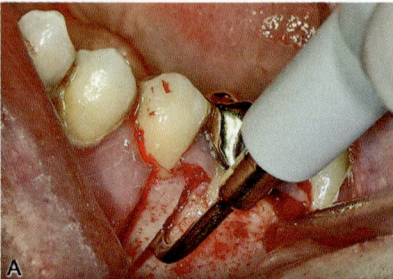

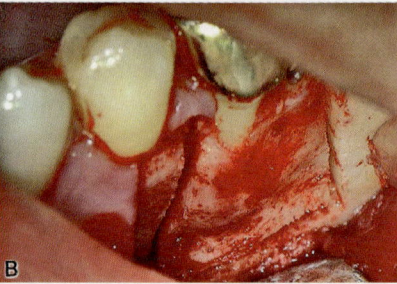

Piezosurgery system:
A. Main unit with panel (I), peristaltic pump (II), socket for connector to handpiece (III); B. Handpiece with saw insert.

Osteotomy being performed using piezoelectric unit

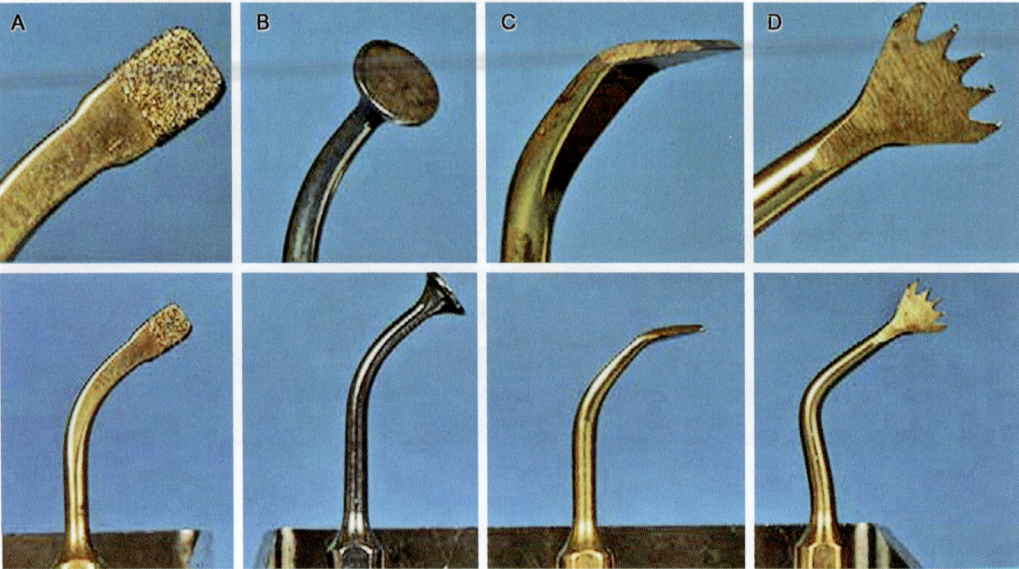

Piezosurgery insert:
A. Flat scalpel, diamond tipped, titanium nitride-coated surface;   B. Cone compressor, flat, blunt;
C. Bone harvester, titanium nitride-coated surface;   D. Sharp tipped saw, titanium nitride-coated surface

Equipment

1. A main unit.
2. Piezoelectric handpiece.
3. A foot switch connected to a main unit.
4. Tooltips called "inserts".

Working Mechanism

Piezosurgery utilizes microvibrations for cutting bone. These are created by the piezoelectric effect: Certain ceramics and crystals deform when an electric current is passed across them, resulting in oscillations of ultrasonic frequency. The settings of power and frequency modulation of the device can be selected on a control panel with a digital display and a keypad according to the planned task. The unit uses a frequency of 25–29 kHz. In boosted mode, a digital modulation of this oscillation produces an alteration of high frequency vibrations with pauses at a frequency of up to 30 kHz. This alteration prevents the insert from impacting the bone and avoids overheating while maintaining optimum cutting capacity. The piezoelectric inserts move between 60 and 120 μm.

Indications

Piezoelectric unit is used to perform bone cutting or osteotomy in:
- Third molar surgery and sinus lift operations.
- Bone biopsies and bone graft harvesting.
- Orthognathic surgery to perform osteotomies.

ROBOTICS FOR SURGERY

Robotic technology is enhancing surgery through improved precision, stability, and dexterity. In image-guided procedures, robots use magnetic resonance and computed tomography image data to guide instruments to the treatment site. This requires new algorithms and user interfaces for planning procedures; it also requires sensors for registering the patient's anatomy with the preoperative image data. Minimally invasive procedures use remote controlled robots that allow the surgeon to work inside the organ.

Information flow in robotic systems for minimally invasive surgery. The surgeon moves the master manipulators; these motions are sent as position commands to the robotic instruments that manipulate tissues within the patient's body. The surgeon views the internal operative field through video images from an endoscope, which is manipulated by another robotic system. Some systems also furnish audio, force, or tactile information.

Strengths

- Good geometric accuracy, stable and untiring.
- Can be designed for a wide range of scales and may be sterilized.
- Resistant to radiation and infection.
- Can use diverse sensors (chemical, force, acoustic, etc.) in control.

Limitations

- Poor judgment.
- Limited dexterity and hand-eye coordination.

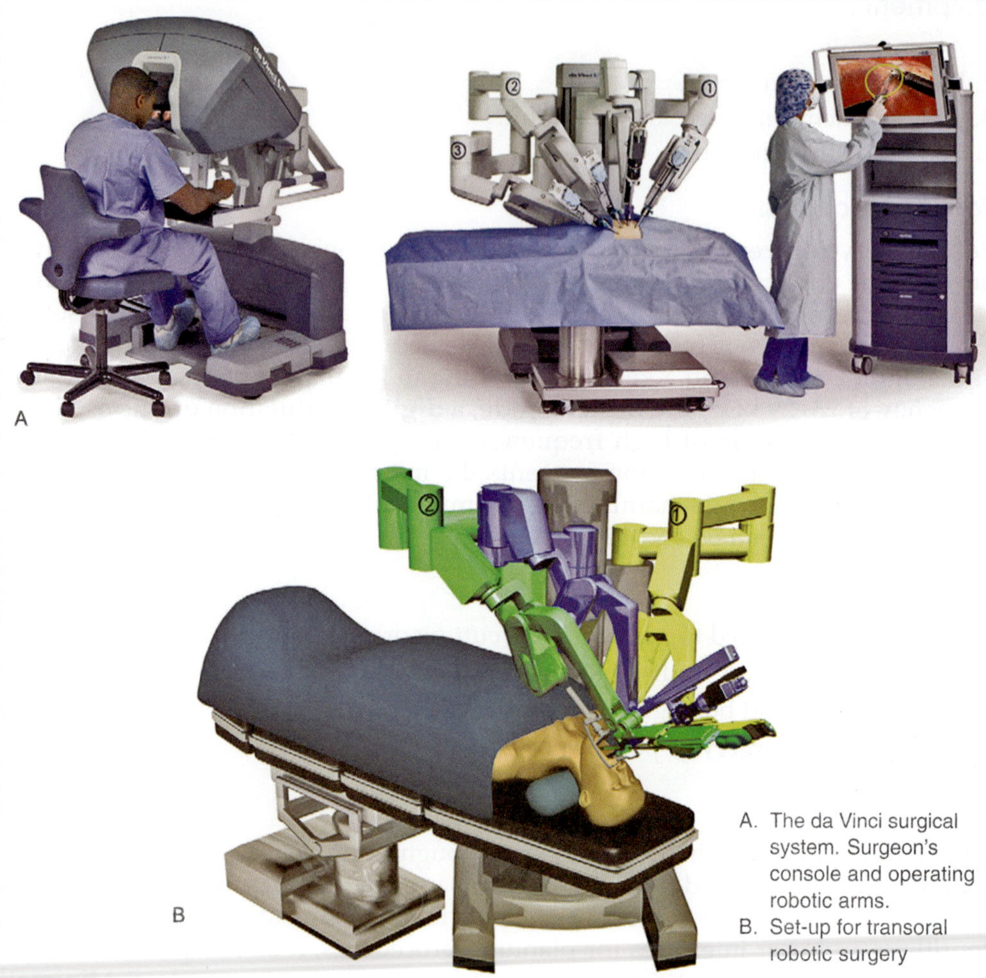

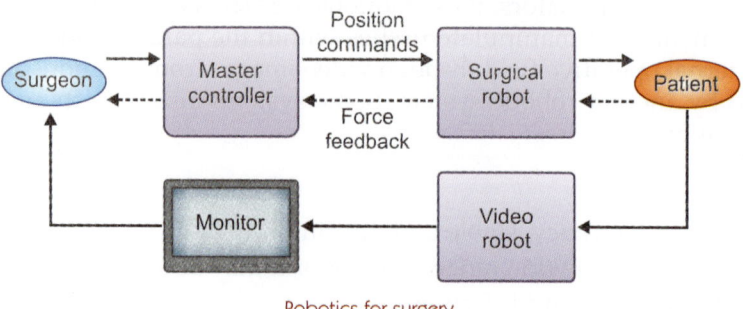

A. The da Vinci surgical system. Surgeon's console and operating robotic arms.
B. Set-up for transoral robotic surgery

Robotics for surgery

- Limited to relatively simple procedures.
- Expensive.
- Technology in flux and difficult to construct and debug.

Bibliography

1. Biohorizons Company Pvt. Ltd. External Implant System Catalogue 2015.

2. Daniel M Laskin. Instruments used in American oral and maxillofacial surgery. J Oral and Maxillofac Surg. 2015;73 (6) :1181 e1-1181 –e6.

3. Georg Eggers, Johannes Klein, Julia Blank, Stefan Hassfeld. Piezosurgery: an ultrasound device for cutting bone and its use and limitations in maxillofacial surgery.Br J Oral Maxillofac Surg. 2004;42(5):451–3.

4. Gvalani AK: Manual of Instruments and Operative Surgery. 1st ed. New Delhi: CBS Publishers.

5. http//en.wikipedia.org/wiki/surgical instrument.

6. http://en.wikipedia.org/wiki/sushruta_samhita.

7. John Kirkup. The history and evolution of surgical instruments. Ann R Coll Surg Engl 1995; 77:386–8.

8. KLS Martin Group company catalogue, Distraction product overview.

9. Perenack JD. The endoscopic brow lift. Atlas Oral Maxillofac Surg Clin North Am. 2016; 24(2): 165–73.

10. Robert D. Howe, Yoky Matsuokas. Robotics for Surgery Annu. Rev. Biomed. Eng. 1999. 01: 211–40.

11. Robert M. Kellman. Endoscopic Craniomaxillofacial Surgery. Facial plastic Surgery Clin of North Am Feb 2008; Vol.14. No. 1.

12. Selective images from internet source

13. SK Surgical Instruments Catalogue, Pune, Maharashtra.

14. VS Arora, Arun Yadav. Synopsis of medical instruments and procedures, 1st ed. pp. 225–71.

Index